Lecture Notes of the Institute for Computer Sciences, Social Informatics and Telecommunications Engineering 359

José Antonio Marmolejo-Saucedo ·
Pandian Vasant · Igor Litvinchev ·
Roman Rodriguez-Aguilar ·
Felix Martinez-Rios (Eds.)

Computer Science and Health Engineering in Health Services

4th EAI International Conference, COMPSE 2020
Virtual Event, November 26, 2020
Proceedings

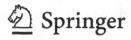 Springer

Editors
José Antonio Marmolejo-Saucedo Ⓘ
Facultad de Ingeniería
Universidad Panamericana
Mexico City, Mexico

Pandian Vasant Ⓘ
Faculty of Science and Information
Technology
Universiti Teknologi Petronas
Teronoh, Perak, Malaysia

Igor Litvinchev Ⓘ
Universidad Autónoma de Nuevo León
San Nicolás de los Garza, Nuevo León,
Mexico

Roman Rodriguez-Aguilar Ⓘ
Ciencias Económicas y Empresariales
Universidad Panamericana
Benito Juárez, Mexico

Felix Martinez-Rios Ⓘ
Facultad de Ingeniería
Universidad Panamericana
Ciudad de México, Mexico

ISSN 1867-8211   ISSN 1867-822X (electronic)
Lecture Notes of the Institute for Computer Sciences, Social Informatics
and Telecommunications Engineering
ISBN 978-3-030-69838-6   ISBN 978-3-030-69839-3 (eBook)
https://doi.org/10.1007/978-3-030-69839-3

This Springer imprint is published by the registered company Springer Nature Switzerland AG
The registered company address is: Gewerbestrasse 11, 6330 Cham, Switzerland

Preface

Once again, we are pleased to present to you the proceedings of the EAI International Conference on Computer Science and Engineering in Health Services (COMPSE). This year, due to global travel problems due to the COVID-19 pandemic, the conference took place virtually, coordinated from Mexico City, Mexico.

The participation of people from various countries was enriching for the general audience. COMPSE brought together research scientists, decision-makers, managers, executives, engineers, academicians, and practicing researchers around the world who are leveraging and developing research in the fields of engineering, computing, health systems, and applied mathematics.

All of them daily face various complex real-world problems and develop and use powerful intelligent computational techniques to solve them. For this reason, the EAI International Conference on Computer Science and Engineering in Health Services (COMPSE 2020) highlights the latest research innovations and applications of algorithms designed for optimization applications within the fields of Science, Computer Science, Engineering, Information Technology, Economics, and Health Systems.

On this occasion, the keynote lecture was given by Prof. Tatiana Romanova from the Department of Mathematical Modeling and Optimal Design at the A. Podgorny Institute for Mechanical Engineering Problems of the National Academy of Sciences of Ukraine, who presented "The phi-function technique and its applications in additive manufacturing". We appreciate the valuable participation of Prof. Romanova and her lecture on novel approaches to optimization in packaging problems.

The 4th EAI International Conference on Computer Science and Engineering in Health Services 2020 received 39 submitted papers of which 16 full papers were accepted and presented. The technical program was arranged into the following tracks: Track 1 – New approaches to supply chain modeling; Track 2 – Health systems: Strategies for the delimitation of vulnerable areas and identification of failures of medical equipment; Track 3 – Applied optimization; and Track 4 – Applications in the education sector.

Coordination with the steering chairs, Prof. Imrich Chlamtac, Prof. Pandian Vasant, and Prof. Igor Litvinchev, was essential for the success of the conference. We sincerely appreciate their constant support and guidance. I also thank Profs. Roman Rodriguez, Utku Köse and Félix Martínez for their collaboration as General Co-Chairs of this edition of the conference. Their excellent work was very important to reach the audience obtained. It was also a great pleasure to work with such an excellent organizing committee team for their hard work in organizing and supporting the conference. In particular, the Technical Program Committee, led by our TPC Chair, Prof. Jania Saucedo, completed the peer-review process of technical papers and made a high-quality technical program. Finally, we are also grateful to our Conference

Manager, Natasha Onofrei, for her constant support and to all the authors who submitted their papers to COMPSE 2020.

José Antonio Marmolejo-Saucedo

Conference Organization

Steering Committee

Imrich Chlamtac	Bruno Kessler Professor, University of Trento, Italy
Pandian Vasant	University Teknologi PETRONAS, Malaysia
Igor Litvinchev	Autonomous University of Nuevo León, Mexico

Organizing Committee

General Chair

José Antonio Marmolejo-Saucedo	Universidad Panamericana Mexico

General Co-chairs

Roman Rodriguez	Universidad Panamericana, Mexico
Igor Litvinchev	Autonomous University of Nuevo León, Mexico
Pandian Vasant	Universiti Teknologi PETRONAS, Malaysia
Utku Köse	Süleyman Demirel University,Turkey
Félix Martínez	Universidad Panamericana, Mexico

TPC Chair and Co-chair

Jania Saucedo	Universidad Autónoma de Nuevo León, Mexico

Sponsorship and Exhibit Chair

Alfonso Murillo Suárez	Universidad Panamericana, Mexico

Local Chair

Alejandro Ordoñez	Universidad Panamericana, Mexico

Workshops Chair

Alfonso Murillo Suárez	Universidad Panamericana, Mexico

Publicity and Social Media Chair

Johanna Bolaños Zúñiga	Autonomous University of Nuevo León, Mexico

Publications Chair

Jania Saucedo	Universidad Autónoma de Nuevo León, Mexico

Web Chair

Alfonso Murillo Suárez   Universidad Panamericana, Mexico

Technical Program Committee

Oliverio Cruz Mejía   Autonomous University of Mexico State, Mexico
Monica Chis   Freelance, Romania
Ugo Fiore   University of Naples Federico II, Italy
Bharat Singh   Nomad Digital GMBH, Germany
Warusia Yassin   Technical University of Malaysia Malacca, Malaysia
Majdi Quttainah   Kuwait University, Kuwait
Dadmehr Rahbari   TalTech, Estonia
Nuno Pombo   University of Beira Interior, Portugal
Esko Turunen   Tampere University, Finland
Bruno Silva   IADE-Universidade Europeia; Universidade da Beira
                             Interior, Portugal
Rustem Popa   "Dunărea de Jos" University of Galaţi, Romania
Zeya Oo   Yangon Technological University, Myanmar
John Escobar   Pontifical Xavierian University, Colombia
Abdellah Derghal   LGEA Laboratory, Algeria
Rosana Cavalcante de   Embrapa, Brazil
  Oliveira
Ömer Deperlioğlu   Afyon Kocatepe University, Turkey
Jude Hemanth   Karunya University, India
Socorro Rangel   São Paulo State University, Brazil
Bhupesh Singh   G.B. Pant University of Agriculture and Technology,
                             India
Ankur Bist   KIET Ghaziabad, India
J. Joshua Thomas   UOW Malaysia KDU Penang University College,
                             Malaysia

Contents

Applied Optimization

Applications in the Education Sector

New Approaches to Supply Chain Modeling

Classification and Clustering of Clients of a Company Dedicated to the Distribution of Auto Parts in the Metropolitan Area of Monterrey

Leonardo G. Hernández Landa[✉] ⓘ, Rosa E. Mata Martinez,
Argelia Vargas Moreno ⓘ, and Arlethe Y. García Aguilar ⓘ

Facultad de Ciencias Químicas, Universidad Autónoma de Nuevo León,
66647 Monterrey, NL, Mexico
leonardo.hernandezln@uanl.edu.mx

Abstract. In this research work, we have collaborated with a company with a local presence dedicated to the sale and distribution of auto parts. The main problem is the lack of an optimized system of distribution to customers, which is capable of accelerating the delivery process. Particularly in this work, we have developed a method to calculate the correct clustering of customers by areas considering the density and volume of order. The result is a classification and assignment of a zone to each customer by the method of k-medoid considering two measures of performance of the literature in order to take the best.

Keywords: Clustering · Level of service · Logistics

1 Introduction

The study was conducted in a company dedicated to the sale and distribution of automotive parts, this company has positioned itself in the domestic market with 11 branches strategically located in Culiacan, Guadalajara, Mexico City, Merida, Monterrey, Puebla, Villahermosa, Tampico, Toluca, and Leon Guanajuato. This company is one of the most important auto parts wholesalers in Mexico, serving more than 7,000 automotive parts stores throughout the country.

In the city of Monterrey N.L. this company is one of the main wholesalers and they are looking to consolidate as the biggest supplier of the city based on their growth strategy.

Excellence in the Supply Chain is pursued, a fundamental part of customer service is efficiency in the delivery of purchase orders to customers. In the Monterrey branch, delivery is made employing different types of fleet. It has pick-up trucks, motorcycles, and cars that distribute throughout the Monterrey metropolitan area and in cities within its coverage area.

J. A. Marmolejo-Saucedo et al. (Eds.): COMPSE 2020, LNICST 359, pp. 3–11, 2021.
https://doi.org/10.1007/978-3-030-69839-3_1

The company seeks to define the best distribution alternative that will improve delivery times and take advantage of the resources it currently has adequately and sustainably.

The project has three main stages, which are listed below, and the process is detailed.

- First stage. Analysis of the current state of the distribution system and classification of customers.
- Second stage. Analysis of distribution alternatives and development of distribution algorithms.
- Third stage. Control and improvement.

1.1 Literature Review

The central feature of the old economy was the mass production and consumption of commodities. The modern economy is based on the production and consumption of increasingly differentiated goods and services [1]. [2] point out in their findings that the value of a service product is largely defined by perceptions of quality. Therefore, service consumers seem to place more importance on the quality of a service than on the costs associated with its acquisition. [3] in her research determines that service quality acts on service loyalty through customer satisfaction.

On the subject of distribution [4] suggest that clients evaluate the process of placing an order by considering the design, information accuracy, privacy, functionality and ease of use of a system. The quality of this process, in turn, positively affects their perceptions of the quality of the transaction outcome. The quality of the transaction outcome subsequently affects satisfaction evaluations. In the case of a problem, the way the retailer handles service recovery has a positive impact on satisfaction, and satisfaction measured the relationship from recovery and quality of results to purchase intentions. [5] in his exploration finds that service quality improvement initiatives must begin with defining customer needs and preferences, and their related quality dimensions.

That is why the first stage begins with the analysis of customer behavior, the value chain and thus finding the most important parameters and variables to establish the appropriate model. The classification of clients by location is one of the techniques that are used to make a correct routing of vehicles for the distribution of products.

[6] developed a cost estimation based on clustering to facility location and demonstrate the first step is to have an adequate technique for classifying clients through their geographic location, access, concentration and importance.

[7] performs a classification using data mining such that it identifies the high-profit, high-value and low-risk customers. [8] optimize the distribution of products with drones, the first step is to classify clients partitioning of delivery locations into small clusters, identifying a focal point per cluster, and routing through all focal points.

2 Methodology

2.1 Analysis of the Current State of the Service

The Monterrey branch currently has a portfolio of approximately 400 clients of which more than 250 have regular activity. Most of the clients' activities are not constant, however the recurrent clients are frequent. Figure 1 shows that the 10 clients with the highest participation represent 32.4% of the total activity, the 20 most frequent clients represent 45% of the activity and the 50 most frequent clients represent 63% of the total activity.

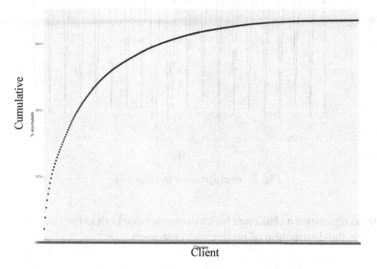

Fig. 1. Accumulated activity by client

The average daily activity per customer is 5 lines, you can see in Fig. 2. The average number of orders processed by the branch is 150 per working day, and in Fig. 3 it can be seen that demand is maintained on working days at high peaks. This results in an average of 700 to 800 products being shipped per day in the week.

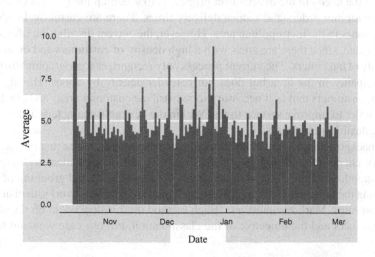

Fig. 2. Average number of products ordered per day per customer

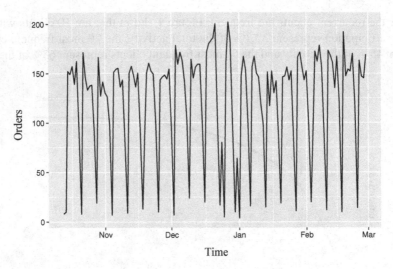

Fig. 3. Average order trend per day

This trend represents a challenge for customer service both in the internal warehouse process and in the distribution of products to customers.

2.2 Classification and Clustering

The actual process starts with the generation of a purchase order, the product stock is checked in the system, consequently the purchase order is passed to the warehouse department to collect the product, the order invoice is generated, it is assigned to a driver for distribution together with other purchase orders and finally it is delivered to the customer in route.

One of the needs in the distribution process is to speed up the process of assigning routes to customer orders and reduce delivery times. There are currently 11 identified customer zones in the metropolitan area. However, the current distribution of customers is not adequate, since there are areas with a high density of customers and others with a low density of customers. The current process only recognizes a geographic distribution per municipality in the area but does not consider density by zones. Having a large number of customers makes it necessary to redistribute customer areas and create better routes in order to improve service times. Within the desirable characteristics is that it is dynamic, flexible and precise.

As a background there are many works in the scientific literature that have managed to classify clients through the use of data analysis and mathematical techniques. [9] make a compilation until 2009 of the methods of classification and grouping of clients, highlighting the most used techniques among which are neural networks, decision trees, association rules, Markov chains, etc. Each method used is dependent on the structure of the customers and the objective of the classification. For our case we want to group the customers based on the following aspects: Geographic location, sales volume, geographic dispersion and workload balancing for the fleet. In [10] a complete guide to geospatial information management in points of interest is presented.

A collection of the precise geospatial information of the customers is made in order to analyze their location and visualize the distribution challenge. Figure 4 shows only the main customers distributed throughout the city of Monterrey and its metropolitan area.

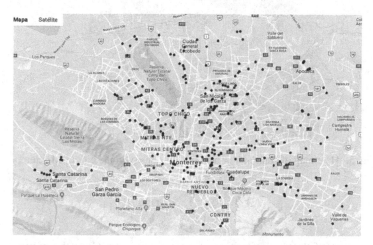

Fig. 4. Physical location of the clients of the Monterrey branch

At first glance, the density of the client concentration is not noticeable, since the concentration of the dots is lost in the dotted display, so Fig. 5 shows the heat map where the green color represents a higher degree of client concentration and is degraded to purple. Greater concentration is observed in the central zone of the municipality of Monterrey and in the central zone of the municipality of San Nicolas de los Garza. The center of Santa Catarina, Apodaca and Guadalupe also show a higher intensity with respect to the rest of the metropolitan area. It can be seen how the municipality of Santa Catarina is separated from the density map and it is important to take this into account when making the classification.

For the clustering of clients, it is decided to use the partition around the medoids with estimation of the number of groups. The method is described in [11] where k representative objects, called medoids (selected from the data set) are searched for that can serve as *prototypes.* for the group instead of the means to allow the use of other arbitrary dissimilarities and arbitrary input domains, using the absolute error criterion (Total deviation) as a target.

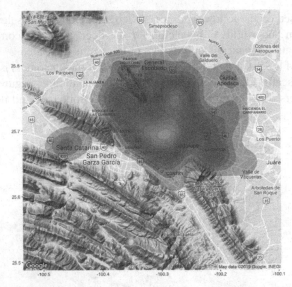

Fig. 5. Heat map of customer concentration density in the city of Monterrey

$$TD := \sum_{i=1} \sum_{x_j \in C_i} d\left(x_j, m_i\right)$$

which is the sum of the dissimilarities of each point $x_j \in C_i$ to the medoid of each cluster. If we use the Euclidean squared distance function (i.e., $d(x, m) = |x - m|_2^2)$,), we almost get the usual SSQ target used by k-means, except that k-medoids is free to choose any $\mu_i \in \mathbb{R}^d$, while in k-median $m_i \in C_i$ must be one of the original data points.

For Euclidean squared distances and Bregman divergences, the arithmetic mean is the optimal choice for μ and a fixed group assignment. For distance L_1 (that is, $\sum |x_i - y_i|$), also called Manhattan distance, the median of the components is a better choice. The medoid of a C set is defined as the object with the smallest sum of differences (or, equivalently, the smallest average) from all other objects in the set

$$\text{medoid}(C) := \arg\min \sum_{x_i \in C} d\left(x_i, x_j\right)$$

the "Partition Around Medoids" (PAM) algorithm consists of two phases, one of construction and another of improvement by means of exchange that optimizes the grouping. It should be noted that this algorithm works on $O(k)$.

For this article we consider the performance measures: Average silhouette width ASW [12] and [13] index CH.

ASW and CH attempt to balance a small within-cluster heterogeneity (which increases) and a large between-cluster heterogeneity (which increases with k as well) in a supposedly optimal way [14].

3 Results

The clustering algorithm is executed on a computer with an Intel core i5 processor with 6 GB of RAM. The development of the cleaning, selection and classification algorithm is executed in the R language, creating a variation of clustering scenarios of the customers to verify the sensitivity of the algorithm to reclassify the groups in cases of fleet size change or the generation of a new clustering strategy. Instances from 4 clusters up to 20 clusters were executed in order to analyze the different alternatives and reach a conclusion on how many clusters for the client classifications are necessary.

As you can see in Table 1 the best metrics are between 9 and 12 clusters according to the AWS and CH metrics. That directly adjusts to the size of the fleet of vehicles that the company has to carry out the delivery of the products.

Table 1. Results by number of cluster VS performance measures

Number of clusters	ASW	CH
4	0.3923259	190.9851
5	0.3856825	198.5562
6	0.3662694	186.4601
7	0.3674657	191.7803
8	0.3857323	192.7776
9	0.3582335	183.0448
10	0.3995877	184.6448
11	0.3812556	176.7437
12	0.3740707	174.2456
13	0.3810907	172.2084
14	0.3942427	184.6819
15	0.4011587	181.5634
16	0.4085602	184.3999
17	0.4145238	255.751
18	0.4040372	254.3008
19	0.414239	261.3025
20	0.4102043	260.5144

Figure 6 is the final result of grouping customers by the available fleet as can be seen in the colors so that the supplier can find a better way to order and make the process much faster.

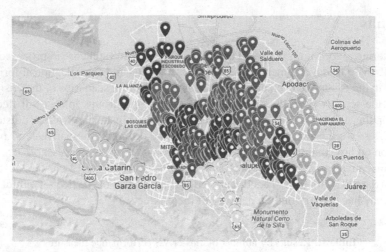

Fig. 6. Final grouping with 11 client clusters

4 Discussion and Further Work

After the analysis, a methodology was established for the classification and grouping of clients for stage one of the projects. The final document provided to the company is a database supported with google maps so they can manipulate the details of each client and create a better routing. The result will speed up the process of route generation and distribution of products in order to reduce loading time. In the same way, this classification will allow the generation of optimal routes for the distribution units, since a lower sectorization will allow to speed up the route search algorithms when considering smaller groups of customers. The efficiency of the algorithm was demonstrated by maintaining the level of homogeneity in the variation of the number of clusters and it is expected that in the future the level of activity of the customer will be introduced to improve the algorithm.

References

1. Fornell, C., Johnson, M.D., Anderson, E.W., et al.: The American customer satisfaction index: nature, purpose, and findings. J. market. **60**(4), 7–18 (1996)
2. Cronin, J.J., Brady, M.K., Tomas, G., Hult, M.: Assessing the effects of quality, value, and customer satisfaction on consumer behavioral intentions in service environments. J. Retail. **76**, 193–218 (2000)
3. Caruana, A.: Service loyalty Service loyalty the effects of service quality and the mediating role of customer satisfaction. Eur. J. Mark. **36**, 309–0566 (2002). https://doi.org/10.1108/030 90560210430818
4. Collier, J., Bienstock, C.: Measuring service quality in e-retailing. Artic J. Serv. Res. (2006). https://doi.org/10.1177/1094670505278867

5. Yang, Z., Kim, D., Jun, M., Kong, H.: Customers' perceptions of online retailing service quality and their satisfaction Implementation of a cross-border charity project: institutional distance partnership arrangement and project performance view project customers' perceptions of online retailing service quality and their satisfaction. Artic Int. J. Qual. Reliab. Manag. (2004). https://doi.org/10.1108/02656710410551728

6. Klose, A., Klose, A.: Using Clustering Methods in Problems of Combined Location and Routing. https://doi.org/10.1007/978-3-642-80117-4_71

7. Rajagopal, S.: Customer data clustering using data mining technique. Int. J. Database Manag. Syst. (IJDMS 3) (2011). https://doi.org/10.5121/ijdms.2011.3401

8. Salama, M., Srinivas, S.: Joint optimization of customer location clustering and drone-based routing for last-mile deliveries. Transp. Res. Part C Emerg. Technol. **114**, 620–642 (2020). https://doi.org/10.1016/j.trc.2020.01.019

9. Ngai, E.W.T., Xiu, L., Chau, D.C.K.: Application of data mining techniques in customer relationship management: a literature review and classification. Expert Syst. Appl. **36**, 2592–2602 (2009)

10. Baddeley, A., Rubak, E., Turner, R., et al.: Spatial Point Patterns. Chapman and Hall/CRC (2015)

11. Schubert, E., Rousseeuw, P.J.: Faster k-Medoids Clustering: Improving the PAM, CLARA, and CLARANS Algorithms (2018)

12. Van der Laan, M.J., Pollard, K.S., Bryan, J.: A new partitioning around medoids algorithm. J. Stat. Comput. Simul. **73**, 575–584 (2003). https://doi.org/10.1080/0094965031000136012

13. Caliński, T., Harabasz, J.: A dendrite method foe cluster analysis. Commun. Stat. **3**, 1–27 (1974). https://doi.org/10.1080/03610927408827101

14. Hennig, C., Liao, T.F.: How to find an appropriate clustering for mixed-type variables with application to socio-economic stratification. J. R. Stat. Soc. Ser. C (Appl. Stat.) **62**, 309–369 (2013). https://doi.org/10.1111/j.1467-9876.2012.01066.x

Guide for Sustainable Project Analysis
to Improve Energy Efficiency of Mexican SME

Luz María Adriana Reyes Ortega[1]([⊠]) [iD] and Román Rodríguez Aguilar[2] [iD]

[1] Universidad Anáhuac, Av Universidad Anáhuac 46, 52786 Naucalpan de Juarez, Mexico
adrianareyeso@hotmail.com
[2] Facultad de Ciencias Económicas Y Empresariales, Universidad Panamericana,
Augusto Rodin 498, 03920 Ciudad de Mexico, Mexico
rrodrigueza@up.edu.mx

Abstract. Faced with the need of overall cleaner production processes, the Government of Mexico, in coalition with international cooperation agencies, has made efforts to spark to a cleaner transition by the conferment of financing under preferential conditions for small and medium-sized enterprises (SMEs), which are the backbone of the Mexican economy. This will help the implementation of sustainable projects that promote the reduction of energy consumption and Greenhouse Gas (GHG) emissions. However, these efforts have not yielded the expected results since the viability of the loans is determined by the Financial Institutions (FIs) based solely on profitability analysis of the SMEs. If this analysis is complemented with consideration of environmental and social aspects, a greater number of projects would be subject to financing. Real Options method allows the calculation of future cash flows incorporating the uncertainty from the volatility associated with the projects, allowing future adjustments to be made to them based on their performance. In addition, under the economic cost-effectiveness analysis, costs incurred in the implemented projects are compared against the results, assigning a monetary value to them to determine their overall impact. Derived from the limitations in the valuation of sustainable projects in SMEs, this article aims to establish a guide for comprehensive evaluation, using a cost-effectiveness approach and addressing the uncertainty of the project through Real Options. Considering the diversity of the SME during this study, the target companies and the type of projects that have the best opportunities for successful application of the proposed guide were segmented.

Keywords: Sustainable financing · SMEs · Real Options · Cost-effectiveness

1 Introduction

In recent years, Mexico's Small and Medium Enterprises (SMEs) Programs have been implemented to motivate the adoption of renewable energies for their operations or placement of energy efficiency measures to reduce their energy consumption, and at the same time, improve their financial profitability. An example is the Introduction Project to

J. A. Marmolejo-Saucedo et al. (Eds.): COMPSE 2020, LNICST 359, pp. 12–30, 2021.
https://doi.org/10.1007/978-3-030-69839-3_2

Energy Efficiency and Energy Management Systems in SMEs in Mexico (2015–2017), which aimed to promote among companies the adoption of energy efficiency practices (through training) and installment of an Energy Management System in each of the participants. 21 companies participated and of these, the Program yielded 17 success stories. Given that there are 4.1 million of these companies, this sample represents a marginal participation [1] of the overall SME universe.

SMEs represent an important energy consumer and consequently, emitters of large concentrations of Greenhouse Gases (GHG) [2]. The Federal Government, with the support of international cooperation agencies [3], Development Banks and specialized entities in sustainable development, has launched financing programs[4] with financial preferential conditions (compared to those offered in the market) that seek to raise awareness among entrepreneurs and business owners about investing in a "sustainable project", that is, in projects that involve investing in energy efficiency or clean energy adoption for their production processes, which in turn will generate savings in their electrical expenses and, in a related way, will generate positive environmental impacts.

As mentioned before, these programs are offered through financing, accompanied by training and technical assistance [4], making up the most efficient approach to potentialize the resources allocated for this objective and enhances the number of beneficiaries.

Yet, the main obstacle to measuring their true impact is that, so far, the only metric in which the results of these projects are evaluated in SMEs is through profitability, since the Financial Institutions (FIs), mainly Banks, do credit management.

In parallel, those involved in promoting sustainable projects to SMEs do not have the necessary elements to test the comprehensive impacts of these projects, whose results are of interest to international organizations. If there were an efficient record of positive impacts generated by these projects, through financial cooperation mechanisms (donations, grants, very low-cost loans), the granting of resources from these organizations could be triggered at a low fundraising cost, and thus strengthen the national portfolio of actions carried out in matters of sustainability.

The resources granted by international organizations make the lending conditions offered for this purpose more attractive since they achieve better interest rates, terms, and larger amounts. This translates into SMEs transforming their production processes into cleaner methods, with better production practices and enhanced commercialization. If the evaluation is limited only to financial factors, the implementation of these projects will continue to be slow and low impact because there is a lack of evidence to verify that their impacts are beyond economic.

Real options have been used since the 70s to evaluate projects under high degrees of uncertainty, having as an initial precedent the study by Black and Scholes [5] and later, presented in a simpler way, the contribution of Cox, Ross and Rubinstein [6]. But it was until 1985, that Brennan and Schwartz [7] evaluated a project on natural resources, which by their nature, have a high degree of uncertainty in pricing. In their work they considered the options of opening, closing, and abandoning the operations of a copper mine, as well as the price of each alternative. Trigeorgis and Mason [8] analyzed different types of projects with real options and were able to demonstrate that the options to reduce, expand or close natural resource projects depend directly on the variation in the prices of the assets or the added value of the project.

Also, there are studies where Real Options have been used for the evaluation of companies and projects, such as "Valuation by Real Options. Theories and cases" [9], where it is precisely proposed how to calculate the value of a company under this method. The article concludes that the information provided by the traditional Net Present Value (NPV) model is not enough to calculate the real value of the company. Real Option analysis complements the valuation beyond cashflow analysis and monetizes sustainability factors for an overall result.

Regarding the cost-effectiveness analysis, this guide parts from the results obtained in the evaluation of Chávez, Gómez, and Briseño [10], where this type of analysis is used as a tool to choose the best option in various possible scenarios. The study also was carried out in a situation where there is interest in reducing GHG emissions. In the same way, in the analysis by Prieto L. [11] the methodology was detailed to select the most suitable scenario among several options with similar characteristics but identifying the best cost-effective option.

2 Background

The SMEs are commonly called the backbone of the Mexican economy since there are about 4.1 million companies. They employ 72% of the total workforce and contribute 52% to the country's Gross Domestic Product [12].

But likewise, the main source of electricity for these SMEs is generation by burning hydrocarbons, which generates enormous amounts of GHG. Thus, in recent years, the Mexican Government has launched programs focused on energy efficiency measures in SMEs and aim to mitigate the effects of climate change, focused on energy efficiency measures in SMEs and seek to reduce the current demand for fossil fuel electricity production in Mexico. Their use generates over 60% of the total GHG emissions and more than three-quarters of carbon dioxide equivalent emissions (CO_{2e}), according to the 2017 National Energy Balance prepared by the Energy Minister (SENER) [13].

2.1 Energy Consumption of SMEs and Their GHG Emissions

The productive activity of SMEs is also reflected in the consumption of electricity and the demand for hydrocarbons. SMEs are responsible for 17% of the country's total energy consumption (electrical and thermal energy) and 12% of the total Greenhouse Gas emissions generated in Mexico, with a potential total reduction of close to 6.91 million tons of CO_{2e} per year [14].

According to the International Energy Agency (IEA), in Mexico the total electricity consumption in 2016 was 280.62 TW/h [15]. According to the Energy Regulatory Commission (CRE), of this consumption, in 2013 only 25.4% was residential demand [16].

2.2 Benefits of Energy Efficiency and Renewable Energy in SMEs

From an energy standpoint, each energy efficiency project implemented in a thermal or electrical consumption system of an SME, can generate average individual savings between 40 and 100 tons of CO_{2e} per year.

Projects that can use the proposed guidance could reduce 360,000 tons of CO_{2e}/y [14], since they are considered projects that require an energy diagnosis prepared by a consultant, which may involve more than one technology and may involve the modification of the layout of the company or its production processes [17].

From an economic perspective, sustainable projects allow SMEs to generate economic savings in energy consumption. Additionally, companies improve their competitiveness, by implementing sustainable actions that enables low-cost production [17].

2.3 Problems in the Current Evaluation of Sustainable Projects

The way in which sustainable projects are currently being evaluated is not efficient enough because positive (or negative) impact evidence is not extracted and documented. Hence, there´s no information available that demonstrates the comprehensive benefits of their implementation. If data were available, the number of prospects would increase drastically in a domino effect, given demonstrated potential demand (enough interest by the business owner), and more international resources could be accessed, which in turn would improve the financing conditions, ultimately making the projects more profitable and attractive, which is enough motivation to entrepreneurs, business owners and FIs.

This guide addresses the problem directly by helping quantify the environmental and financial criteria and see if combined are enough to incur in financing costs and implementation measures.

3 Methodology

For years, initiatives as the project Introduction to Energy Efficiency and SME Energy Management Systems in Mexico [18], have been launched that promote the transition of the Mexican energy market towards more sustainable production models. The Federal Government has offered subsidies, credits, support with the change of technologies, many of these with the support of international cooperation, new regulations on environmental issues and tax incentives, and despite this, the desired results have not been achieved.

Mexico has international commitments on GHG emissions: reduce 22% of its greenhouse gas emissions by 2030 and 51% with respect to its CO_{2e} emissions [19] but the strategies put in place are still insufficient.

Given that SMEs represent an important consumer of electricity in the country and actively demand resources associated with hydrocarbons, it is necessary to pay attention to the mitigation efforts carried out in this sector.

The number of companies that have adopted a sustainable project can be measured through various programs implemented in the country, as well as their economic profitability, but the real value of these projects, as well as their effectiveness, is uncertain.

For Mexico to continue to be subject of international support, it is necessary to have information tools that can quantify the comprehensive impacts of the implemented projects, with a tangible goal for decision-makers about environmental, social and economic impacts as an integrated objective, making these projects profitable in the process and bringing Mexican SMEs closer to sustainable development.

Additionally, the proposed guide intends to standardize all factors considered when conducting an evaluation of sustainable projects in SMEs, which will serve as a bridge between energy consultants and bank executives to correctly determine the technical and financial viability of these projects.

3.1 Cost-Effectiveness Approach

The Cost-Effectiveness evaluation model is an economic analysis that compares the costs incurred in the implemented projects against their results, assigning a monetary value to their consequences [10].

This evaluation model is useful for social and environmental projects where the impacts do not have an economic value by themselves, but their effects are beneficial for the population and the economy in general.

In the case of evaluating sustainable projects, given the costs of efficient technologies, subsidized electricity rates and the financial situation of SMEs, it is difficult to create profitable projects and, consequently, create lending appetite to FIs for funding. To know its integral value, it is necessary to evaluate its entire process and quantify the positive impacts.

Although knowing the value of these impacts will not automatically make projects attractive for FIs, they will be of interest to the authorities in charge of environmental policies, international cooperation agencies and non-profit associations that can contribute with various incentives to promote the implementation of sustainable projects in SMEs and, consequently, build interest to FIs.

To make economic evaluations under the cost-effectiveness approach, it must be considered that:

The quotient obtained by dividing the net cost of a project by its net benefit or effectiveness is known as "average cost-effectiveness" (CEM). If the result is low, they are cost-effective (efficient) measures, since they have a lower cost for each unit of net benefit or effectiveness that they produce. On the other hand, measures with high CEM are less efficient [11].

When there are several projects that generate benefits, the cost-effectiveness analysis will allow an orderly classification of the relationship between the cost incurred and the effectiveness of the project. For this, the incremental cost-effectiveness (CEI) is used by means of which the costs and effects of the different alternatives are compared, expressed in the same units [11].

The cost-effectiveness plan (see Fig. 1) allows you to place the options, according to their cost and the level of effectiveness. Ideally, the best option is to locate the best project in the second quadrant, where the option is most effective and less expensive.

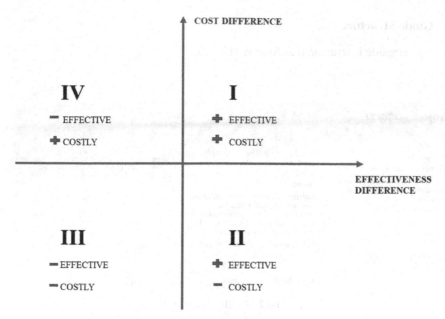

Fig. 1. Cost-effectiveness plan [11].

3.2 Real Options

Real options are a financial instrument that provides the opportunity to make future modifications to a productive project to maximize its value [20]. This tool is useful in sustainable projects due to the high level of uncertainty they have, caused by changes that may occur in the face of technological innovations, price changes and therefore adjustments in the value and profitability of the project that could increase profitability over its operational life.

Real Options allow the investor to make decisions during the life of the project, which add future value and cut losses that a project could incur. With this tool, various actions related to the project can be carried out:

- Expansion or growth: Consider making additional investments related to the project.
- Abandonment: There is the alternative of liquidating the project for another that generates more value for the investor.
- Contraction or reduction: The possibility of reducing the operations related to the project is granted if it is more convenient for the investor.
- Postpone: The project has the option of not executing immediately, since it is estimated that, if expected, the external conditions that affect the project will be more convenient and profitable in the future.
- Flexibility: The investor can change some characteristics of the project during its life continually maximizing its value.

3.3 Guide Structure

The present guide is structured as follows (Fig. 2):

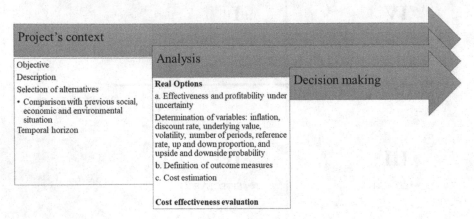

Fig. 2. Guide structure

4 Results

Mexican SMEs consume 43.7% of the national electrical energy, of which 37.3% is demanded by medium-sized companies, which are approximately 400 thousand users and have a saving potential of 11%.

The technologies that present the highest incidence of use in medium-sized companies are electric motors, compressed air systems, lighting, air conditioners, refrigeration, office equipment, and pumping systems. In addition, the installation of photovoltaic solar systems for clean electricity generation is added to activities with potential in energy efficiency. Although there is a clear market segmentation, the implementation of these projects has not been massified because there is a deficiency in the analysis capacity of the projects.

Although a bank credit analyst knows in detail the elements to evaluate the profitability of a project and whether the client is subject to financing, he does not know the technical and environmental particularities that may arise from said project, such as energy savings in fixed expenses, which in turn will increase the borrower's cash flow and increase its debt service payment capacity, nor will it check whether the project will require any modification during its operation cycle to increase its profitability or how cost-effective the project is, by analyzing qualitative and non-quantitative variables.

4.1 Guide Structure

As a result of the evaluation of the proposed methodology, the elements that make up the guide are presented.

Objective. The goal of this guide is to establish a new framework for the evaluation of energy efficiency projects in medium-sized companies, which considers both the profitability of the projects from a Real Options perspective, as well as their results, under a cost-effective approach and thus having a comprehensive perspective of the impacts to the project.

The goal is to increase the number of projects implemented by demonstrating and integrating the associated benefits they generate, besides profitability. To do this, a series of steps are proposed so that decision-makers, in this case, International Cooperation Agencies and FIs, can determine the value of starting a project and decide in which cases is better not to implement it, taking as a reference its financial results and impacts, in a comprehensive manner.

Project Description. To start the evaluation and apply the steps in the guide, data must be gathered that will give the evaluator a complete view of the project. This includes description of stakeholders (SME company name, energy consultant), detailed description of the SME operations and the project to be implemented structuring each energy action or technological change, economic and energy consumption savings, total investment required, Return of Investment, Payback Period, as well as the percentage of efficiency reached by the technologies in their performance.

Additionally, the technical information of the technologies to be implemented is required, as well as knowing the electrical tariff applied the company and the cost per kW/h.

Selection of Alternatives. The results obtained by the implementation of an Energy Efficiency Project in an SME are evaluated against the preconditions in which that company finds itself before the project. Subjects of interest in this guide are projects that have a positive sustainable effect and efficiency, but in some cases are not financially profitable, that is, those projects that provide positive environmental and social impacts, in addition to the profitability sought by Banks.

The comparison will fall mainly in 3 ways:

a. The previous energy consumption of the SME - Environmental aspect.
b. The historical payment of the SME for electricity - Economic aspect.
c. Previous GHG emissions - Social aspect.

These three concepts are integrated to determine if the environmental impact after implementing each project is more sustainable versus the no implementation.

Temporal Horizon. Given that the technologies to be implemented can contemplate useful life cycles of up to 20 years, this period is considered as the guide´s time horizon.

The application of Real Options in the evaluation process seeks to maximize the profitability of projects with interventions over time or minimize losses in case the project does not have a positive performance. Real options contain scenarios under uncertainty, considering the possibility of stopping the project in case of extreme losses or maximize profit if income is higher than expected.

Effectiveness and Profitability Under Uncertainty (Real Options). Traditionally, projects that require financing from Banks are analyzed under the NPV approach, which consists of determining the current value of the project, considering the cashflow generated in the future (applied inflation), by using a discount rate (usually debt interest rate or Weighted Average Cost of Capital) at which the initial investment (equity and/or debt) will be obtained. This method is used in Project Finance practices to determine their added value to shareholders, but it has a deficiency: it does not consider possible changes to the project during its useful life, which could represent maximizing profits or reducing losses.

Starting with the information of the SME and knowing the economic variables of the environment, the cashflow of the company is constructed and the Internal Rate of Return (IRR) is calculated, which determines the percentage of interest that the investment produces. In most cases, the SME does not have the necessary liquidity to implement the project on its own, so an FI is used to request additional funds through debt.

With financing, the initial equity investment is reduced, which causes the IRR of these projects to become more robust. But what if the natural volatility that exists in these projects and / or their associated risks affected their performance? The NPV may not consider it, but the Real Options can.

The Real Options are the result of questioning the traditional method of financial evaluation of a project, where the project is not considered as a static situation. With Real Options, you can calculate future cashflows incorporating the uncertainty from their volatility. Additionally, it considers alternatives for expansion, modification, reduction or closure of the project based in the results it generates over time.

To determine the effectiveness and profitability of a project based on Real Options, it is necessary to determine some variables that describe the particularities of the project, which will allow the construction of the model. These variables are (Table 1):

The Real Options method offers to the traditional evaluation of energy efficiency projects the possibility of determining the present value of future cash flows under conditions of uncertainty, considering the volatility that may exist in them. This uncertainty factor is continuously present in energy efficiency projects as a result of possible 1) technological improvements to the equipment, making the new ones more efficient at a cheaper cost, 2) loss of energy efficiency of the equipment due to any failure, defect or misuse, 3) increases in electricity rates or 4) regulatory changes that do not encourage a cleaner power generation market.

Using the binomial model of Real Options, the initial investment value is calculated before determining the probabilities of raising (up) or lowering (down) the overall value of the project through its life cycle.

The Real Options generate the possibility of evaluating the project at different moments of its productive life, to determine if it is financially convenient to carry out any modification such as expansion, reduction or closure / conclusion of the project.

To estimate the different scenarios, one of the equations must be considered as appropriate (Table 2):

Once the probability that the initial NPV of the project will rise or fall is calculated, using the binomial up-down model, the formula corresponding to each scenario is applied to each probability of year *n* and then all periods are discounted, eliminating the effect of

Table 1. Model variables

Variable	Description
Inflation	Percentage in which prices are generally increased in a unit of time
Discount Rate	Or interest rate, is the cost of capital and / or financing that is used to know the present value of a future flow. It is called r
Underlying Value (S_0)	Present value of cash flows, without discounting the initial investment
Volatility (σ)	Measurement of the frequency and intensity of changes in the value of cash flows (EF) of a project. Is calculated $\sigma = \text{stand.dev.} \sum_{t=1}^{n} ln\left(\frac{EF_t}{EF_{t+1}}\right)$
Number of periods	It is the time that the project will last. A unit of time is defined for its count. It is called n
Reference rate	Also known as the risk-free rate, it is the price paid by risk-free instruments such as Mexican Treasury Bonds (CETES for its name in Spanish), therefore it is compared with the rate of the project, which must be higher than the reference, otherwise it would not have no added value carrying out the project. It is called r_f
Up	It is the proportion of increase expected if the value of the underlying asset increases. Is calculated $u = e^{(\sigma * \sqrt{tvn})}$
Down	It is the proportion of decrease expected if the value of the underlying asset decreases. Is calculated: $d = \frac{1}{u}$
Upside probability	Being a binomial model, it is assumed that the price of the Underlying asset evolves according to a multiplicative binomial process, so that, if the initial price is S_0, in the next period, the price may be $S_0 * u$, with probability p It is calculated as follows: $p = [(1 + r_f) - d]/(u - d)$
Downside probability	If the initial price is S_0, in the next period, the price could be $S_0 * d$, with probability q. Is calculated $q = 1 - p$

the up and down probability and is brought to present value, removing the effect of the interest rate. From the amount obtained, the price of the initial investment is subtracted, and the present value of the project is taken with real options.

The evaluation with real options can give clarity for optimal decision making when faced with the need or desire to modify the original characteristics of the project.

Definition of Outcome Measures. From the financial structure of the project, the environmental factors that are considered as a result measure are determined.

In energy efficiency projects, calculating GHG emissions is relatively simple, since there is an emission factor estimated by the Energy Regulatory Commission (CRE for its acronym in Spanish) which is used to estimate the indirect emissions that come from the use of electricity purchased in the National Electric System (SEN for its acronym in

Table 2. Real Options equations

Type of Option	Value
Option to increase E% by investing I	$FC_t = FC_0 + max(E*FC_0 - I; 0)$
Option to reduce in C%, reducing investment from I1 to I2	$FC_t = MAX(FC_0 - I_1; C * FC_0 - I_2)$
Option to defer or wait a period	$FC_t = MAX(FC_n - I; 0)$
Option to close or abandon with liquidation value	$FC_t = MAX(FC_t; L_t)$
Option of closure or temporary abandonment	$FC_t = MAX(FC_n - cf - cv; E * FC_n - cf)$
Option of selection choice	$FC_t = MAX(E * FC_n - I - C; *FC_n + A; L)$

Spanish). This factor is updated annually because the fuel mix used to generate electricity can vary.

The environmental results measure to be considered in this guide will be the result of multiplying the Emission Factor by the amount of W / h consumed by the company before and after the implementation of the energy efficiency measure.

When comparing the tons of GHG emitted in the initial scenario versus the EE measure scenario, the number of emissions generated should be notably less, so that the project is justified in environmental terms. This measure can represent the added value in projects that have minimum profitability levels, since international cooperation agencies have as their main goal the reduction of GHG emissions, above financial profitability.

Cost Estimation. To determine the costs incurred with the reference measure, that is, emitting or avoiding GHG emissions, it is necessary to relate the cost of producing the MW/h from which the GHGs are emitted.

The first variable that is required to know is the amount of energy required by the company for its activities. The percentage of efficiency that the new equipment will lose is also required to determine the electrical demand that the equipment will have.

It is necessary to multiply the rated power by the productivity of the system and by the efficiency losses that the equipment will have in the first and consecutive years, to obtain the production of electricity that will be obtained through a renewable source of energy. This amount must be multiplied by the emission factor to determine the GHGs generated, considering that these units would have been emitted with a non-sustainable alternative.

To find out the cost of these emissions, the amount of energy produced must be multiplied by the cost of the kW / h that had to be paid to the Mexican Electrical Federal Commission (CFE for its acronym in Spanish and Mexico´s state-owned and main provider of electrical power in the Country) for electricity, affecting said cost with the increase estimate.

Finally, the total cost of electricity is divided by the number of tons of CO_{2e} produced to determine the unit cost per GHG.

The cost per unit indicates what it costs the company to emit each ton of GHG. On the other hand, to determine the positive effect caused by the implementation of an energy efficiency measure, the same amount of GHG is considered but with a negative sign, since they were not emitted and it is divided between the operating and financial expenses in which they are incurred to implement the project.

Any environmental benefit translates into economic benefits for the SME and increases in the value of the implemented project.

Presentation of Results (Cost - effectiveness). Once the results measures and the costs incurred to achieve environmental benefits in the project have been determined, it is necessary to evaluate whether these actions are cost-effective, not only with the initial scenario, but also with other options available in the market, to ensure that the choice made is the best for the company.

To determine which option is the most cost-effective, we must determine the costs associated with the implemented initiative, but also with the elements related to the measurement of results, which is the emission of GHG, its savings and the costs of producing them.

Initially, there must be more than one alternative of efficient equipment to install and that cover the needs of the company. Then, besides to the cost of the equipment, its electrical consumption and the GHG emission of each must be compared to determine which of the options is the most cost-effective. There is equipment that, by its nature, may apparently be more convenient for the company compared to its competition, but in reality it is not, since it may be cheaper, but it is not as efficient, might be very expensive to install or it is very high loss of efficiency over time.

4.2   Case Study

The present guide was used to evaluate two sustainable projects that can be implemented in a SME. The intention of proposing two types of projects is to exemplify that the guide can be used both in large projects that involve the implementation of renewable energies and in simple cases that only involve energy efficiency measures.

The first was the installation of a 352.45 Kilowatt of power (kWp) solar photovoltaic system that would allow the supply of clean electricity to 20 companies in a small industrial complex.

The characteristics of the project are (Table 3):

With the project data, its IRR (21.02%) and NPV ($ 129,811.12) were calculated. The IRR is above the interest rate (15%) and the NPV is positive, which indicates that the investment generates value over time. Since the SME has liquidity problems, it has decided to apply for a bank loan with the following characteristics (Table 4):

Considering financing of 70% of the total investment amount, the IRR increased to 43.88% and the NPV to $ 178,897.28. The IRR increases considerably because the investment generates more value as the initial investment is lower and the NPV is also stronger. But with this information it cannot be determined whether the natural volatility that exists in these projects and / or its associated risks could impact their performance. The NPV may not consider it, but the actual options can. To apply the evaluation using real options, the following values are calculated (Table 5):

Table 3. Project data

Concept	Cost	Unit
Price of plant installations	1,160.00	$/kWp
System rated power	352.45	kWp
Cost of the SSFV	408,842.00	$
1kWp productivity with inverter	1,720.00	kWh/kWp/year
Initial losses in the efficiency of PV modules	1.00	%
Long-term efficiency losses	0.80	% yearly
Self-consumption of the annual production of the plant	100.00	%
Energy cost on the electric bill	0.08	$/kWh
Annual increase in energy cost	5.00	%
Plant life	20	years
Operating costs	25.00	$/kWp/year
Insurance	3.00	$/kWp/year
Inflation	4.00	%
Interest rate or discount	15.00	%
Income Tax	0.00	%

Table 4. Funding conditions

Concept	Cost	Unit
Bank 70%	286,189.40	$
SME Investment 30%	122,652.60	$
Tenor	10	Years

Next, it is evaluated which option could be more profitable, considering the effect of any of the following modifications to the project in an intermediate moment of its useful life, said evaluation was carried out in year 10 under the following scenarios (Tables 6, 7, 8 and 9):

a. Increase the investment amount by 30%, with expenses of 30%.
b. Reduce the investment amount by 25%, with 28% savings.
c. Settle the project with a recovery value of 50%.

With these results, it is concluded that, in year 10, it is not convenient to either reduce the size of the project or liquidate it, but rather expand it, since not only has a bigger NPV, but also the value of the option is positive, indicating that it should be exercised.

Table 5. Project values

Variable	Symbol	Value
Underlying value	S0	$301,549.88
Strike price	I	$122,652.60
Volatility	Σ	67%
Number of periods	N	20 years
Reference rate	rf	7.46%
Up	U	1.9543
Down	D	0.5117
Discount factor	R	1.0746
Upside probability	P	0.3902
Low probability	Q	0.6098

Table 6. Scenarios

Scenarios	Modification
Expansion (E)	30%
Additional investment of 30% (I)	-$ 36,795.78
Shrink (C)	25%
Expected savings of 28% (A)	$ 34,342.73
Settlement value 50% (L)	$ 61,326.30

Table 7. Scenario 1: Increase 30%

Initial NPV	$ 427,471.80
NPV with Real Option	$ 445,391.46
Option Value	$ 17,919.66

Table 8. Scenario 2: Decrease 25%

Initial NPV	$ 422,790.14
NPV with Real Option	$ 243,540.11
Option Value	-$ 179,250.03

Table 9. Scenario 3: Closing with 50% clearance

Initial NPV	$ 415,309.91
NPV with Real Option	$ 302,348.91
Option Value	-$ 112,961.00

In this example, the profit margins are large because we are talking about completely converting the energy supply method, but in energy efficiency projects from other technologies within the target market, the margins are much narrower and the evaluation with Real Options can give us clarity for decision making when faced with the need or desire to modify the original characteristics of the project.

From the financial structure of the project, the environmental factors that are considered as a measure of results are determined.

The environmental results measure considered in this guide will be the result of multiplying the Emission Factor by the amount of Megawatt per hour (MWh) consumed by the company before and after the implementation of the energy efficiency measure. The emission factor that was considered was 0.527 tCO_{2e} / MWh.

When comparing the tons of GHG emitted in both scenarios, the resulting quantity after the implementation of the new technology should be significantly less than the initial figure for the project to be worthwhile in environmental terms. This measure can represent the added value in those projects that have minimum profitability levels, since international cooperation agencies have as their main goal the reduction of GHG emissions, above financial profitability.

To determine the costs incurred with the reference measure, that is, in emitting or avoiding GHG emissions, it is necessary to relate the cost of producing the MW / h from which the GHGs are emitted. This project has the following values (Table 10):

Table 10. Values for GHGs emissions calculation

Concept	Cost	Unit
System rated power	352.45	kWp
1kWp productivity with inverter	1,720.00	kWh/kWp/year
Initial losses in the efficiency of PV modules	1.00	%
Long-term efficiency losses	0.80	% annual
Emission factor	0.527	tCO_{2e} / MWh
Energy cost on the bill	0.08	$/kWh
Annual increase in energy cost	5.00	%

With this, it is determined that the company does not spend more on the emission of GHGs and has savings by not emitting them. At the end of the project's life, about

5,800 tCO$_{2e}$ will have been saved. This environmental benefit translates into economic benefits for the SME and increases the value of the project.

The second model presents a case where a SME wants to replace 2 air conditioning units of 3 tons of refrigeration each, to reduce electricity costs, consumption and the GHG emissions they generate. Both equipment are considered as a replacement option are efficient and meet the needs of the company. The equipment data is as follows (Table 11):

Table 11. Equipment data

Case and costs overview	PAYNE	Mini Split Mirage	Mini Split LG
Description	Initial	Equipment A	Equipment B
Equipment price	$ 18,000.00	$ 23,000.00	$ 28,000.00
Consumption kW / h	37,991.00	27,115.00	33,098.00
Average cost of kW / h	1.89	1.49	1.49
Cost of electricity	$ 71,958.75	$ 40,512.52	$ 49,316.02
Equipment automation cost	$ 199,876.00	$ 151,445.00	$ 151,445.00
Cost of GEI $ / ton CO$_{2e}$	$ 14,476.35	$ 15,042.93	$ 13,115.04
Generated GHG emissions ton CO$_{2e}$	20.02	14.29	17.44

Equipment A is cheaper than equipment B and it generates less GHG emissions. What makes it more cost-effective is that the cost of avoided emissions is lower, so the company will choose equipment A over equipment B (Table 12).

Table 12. Equipment comparison

Cost effectiveness analysis	Equipment A	Equipment B
Equipment costs	$ 214,957.52	$ 228,761.02
Initial equipment costs	$ 289,834.75	$ 289,834.75
Equip. emissions	14.29	17.44
Emissions initial equipment	20.02	20.02
Savings in cost of emissions	**$ 13,063.81**	**$ 23,684.74**

There is equipment that, by its nature, that may apparently be more convenient for the company compared to its competition, but, since there are efficiency issues with use and high installation costs. For this, it is recommended to carry out a cost-effectiveness analysis using as a reference the GHG emissions that will also serve to provide a comparative differentiating element to the available choices.

5 Conclusions

As shown by the results of the Case Study in the present guide, Real Options Cost-effectiveness Analysis are an extremely valuable analytical tools for decision makers that help mitigate uncertainty, while adding versatility for strategic changes that can maximize both profitability and positive environmental impacts. In addition, it also gives a broader perspective beyond the classic financial metrics for credit analysis, and in turn increases lending to sustainable projects.

To summarize, the present guide was applied to test the feasibility of the installation of a 352.45 kWp solar photovoltaic system, and with scenario simulation with Real Options, it was possible to determine that, in year 10 of the project's life, the investment is convenient and the project has GHG savings potential. Likewise, in the case of a SME of replacement of 2 Air Conditioning equipment with 3 Tons of Refrigeration each to reduce its costs for electricity consumption and GHG emissions through the cost effectiveness analysis, it was possible to determine which equipment was the most convenient for both the company and the environment when considering the reduction of tons of GHG that will not be generated.

The world's top economies are gradually moving towards more environmentally friendly production models because of trying to harmonize the economic, social and environmental axes to achieve sustainable growth, with Europe leading as an example. In less developed countries like Mexico, the present guide offers an opportunity to replicate and further incentivize the focus and the benefits of a sustainable perspective to the classic and standard project evaluation; complementing the financial metrics used to assess added value to shareholders. Additional stakeholders (customers, employees, communities) are also considered in this approach, given that the project´s sustainability efforts affect society as a whole and the global environment.

Mexico has carried out actions to integrate this sustainable model to its most significant productive workforce: small and medium enterprises. Yet, the efforts of the Federal Government, international cooperation organizations and specialist entities in sustainability have not been able to achieve the foreseen goals and encourage technological and energy migration towards energy efficiency through financing. This guide not only aims to open new paths of evaluation, but it also helps stakeholders like Mexican financial institutions complement their analysis and have more lending appetite. This in turn can accelerate Mexico´s energetic transition to cleaner sources.

Banks have the enormous challenge of expanding their traditional credit metrics to begin evaluating the integral impacts of the project beyond economic profitability so that, added with the participation of cooperation agencies, access to preferential financing with lower cost and longer term can be achieved, so that the number of benefited SMEs increases and consequently, sustainable development is established in their production processes.

By integrating Real Options in the analysis methodology, as shown before, it also allows close monitoring of projects whose characteristics, given their nature, can be modified throughout their life and, in case of existing financial obligations, during the tenor of the loans. This tool is particularly useful to maximize profits and minimize losses and risks associated with the project, without having to leave aside the non-quantitative elements of the project.

Additionally, the cost-effectiveness evaluation allows the incorporation of qualitative variables, whose result allows the decision maker to carry out a comprehensive review of the impacts of the projects to determine whether, in addition to being financially profitable, it is environmentally viable and positive for society.

Some countries are taking significant action to mitigate Climate Change and its effects, but it's not only up to governments, but professionals as well to help create ways to contribute to the economic system and provide sustainability and clean energy methods to be used in the overall economic infrastructure. This guide provides one perspective that provides reliable qualitative information for decision makers to determine the viability of a sustainable project in an SME and overall, the country.

References

1. CONUEE. https://www.gob.mx/conuee/acciones-y-programas/introduccion-a-la-eficiencia-energetica-y-sistemas-de-gestion-de-energia-en-pymes-de-mexico-pequenas-y-medianas-empresas. Accessed 01 Sept 2020
2. Mexico Government. https://www.gob.mx/cms/uploads/attachment/file/164241/2a_parte.pdf. Accessed 14 Aug 2020
3. Energy Partnership. https://www.energypartnership.mx/es/home/. Accessed 22 Aug 2020
4. Nacional Financiera. https://www.nafin.com/portalnf/files/secciones/financiamiento/fichas_financ/Financiamiento%20sustentable,%20Eco-credito%20empresarial%20masivo.pdf. Accessed 23 Aug 2020
5. Black, F., Scholes, M.: The pricing of options and corporate liabilities. J. Polit. Econ. **81**(3), 637–654 (1973) he University of Chicago Press
6. Cox, J.C., Ross, S.A.: Option pricing: a simplified approach. J. Financ. Econ. **7**, 229–263 (1979)
7. Brenan, M.J., Schwartz, E.S.: Evaluating natural resource investments. J. Bus. **58**(2), 135–157 (1985)
8. Trigeorgis, L., Mason, S.P.: Valuing managerial flexibility'. Midl Corporate Financ. J. **5**(1) 14–21 (1987)
9. Aznar, J., Cayo, T., López, A., Vivancos, J.: Valorazión por opciones reales. Teorias y casos. Universidad Politécnica de Valencia, España (2018)
10. Chávez, C., Gómez, W., Briceño, S. Costo-Efectividad de instrumentos Económicos para el control de la contaminación. El caso del uso de la leña, pp. 197–224. Cuadernos de Economía, Chile (2009)
11. Prieto, L., Sacristán, J., Antoñanzas, F., Rubio-Terrés, C., Pinto, J., Rovira, J.: Análisis coste-efectividad en la evaluación económica de intervenciones sanitarias, pp. 505–510. Med Clin, España (2004)
12. CONDUSEF. https://www.condusef.gob.mx/Revista/index.php/usuario-inteligente/educacion-financiera/492-pymes. Accessed 23 Aug 2020
13. Mexico Government. https://www.gob.mx/cms/uploads/attachment/file/288692/Balance_Nacional_de_Energ_a_2016__2_.pdf. Accessed 03 Sept 2020
14. NAMA Facily. https://www.nama-facility.org/projects/mexico-energy-efficiency-in-smes-as-a-contribution-to-a-low-carbon-economy/. Accessed 17 Aug 2020
15. IEA. https://www.iea.org/countries/Mexico/. Accessed 11 Aug 2020
16. CRE. https://www.cre.gob.mx/documento/3978.pdf. Accessed 10 Aug 2020
17. Iki-Alliance Mexico. https://iki-alliance.mx/download/biblioteca_pronama/nama_pyme/nama_pyme_piloto/GIZ%202013%20Curso%20EE%20PyME%20(NAFIN)%20-%20Gu%C3%ADa.pdf. Accessed 03 Sept 2020

18. CONUEE. https://www.gob.mx/conuee/acciones-y-programas/introduccion-a-la-eficiencia-energetica-y-sistemas-de-gestion-de-energia-en-pymes-de-mexico-pequenas-y-medianas-empresas. Accessed 13 Aug 2020
19. Mexico Government. https://www.gob.mx/inecc/prensa/inecc-reitera-su-compromiso-ante-el-acuerdo-de-paris-con-rutas-de-mitigacion-al-cambio-climatico. Accessed 28 Aug 2020
20. Tresierra Tanaka, Á., Carrasco Montero, C.: Valorización de opciones reales: modelo Ornstein-Uhlenbeck. J. Econ. Financ. Admin. Sci. Peru **21**, 56–62 (2016)

A Multi-product Stochastic Programming Model for Supplier Selection in a Humanitarian Relief Chain

Juan Luis Mejía Miranda$^{(\boxtimes)}$ and Jania Astrid Martínez Saucedo

Faculty of Mechanical and Electrical Engineering, Universidad Autónoma de Nuevo León,
San Nicolas de los Garza, Mexico
{juanluis.mejiamr,jania.saucedomrt}@uanl.edu.mx

Abstract. This paper focuses on the supplier selection in a humanitarian relief chain. Considering the negative impact that natural disasters have in society and their environment, the procurement costs could be a challenging issue for humanitarian organizations (HO). Post-disaster procurement and pre-positioning inventory usually carry large costs due to the haste of the situation in the first or the extensive administration in the latter. This work analyzes supplier selection tools proposed in the literature and focuses primarily on the final decision stage where an organization optimizes the purchase of items from a supplier base.

We propose a scenario-based two-stage stochastic programming model for a statutory agency; it considers a limited budget and the procurement from a higher-level source like the federal government. We also consider framework agreements (FA's) where the buyer commits to purchase some reserved capacity from suppliers during a given period of time (also called horizon) so that better prices could be negotiated and help the organization lower their procurement costs.

The proposed model delivers an optimal solution for a statutory agency and helps in the decision-making process as to what candidate suppliers are desirable to establish a framework agreement with. The solution shows important information as to what percentage of demand is covered from the selected suppliers.

Limited funding in HO's is a very important factor for decision-making. The model incorporates a budget constraint and delivers information about the amount of relief items to procure form a different source other than the supplier base.

Keywords: Humanitarian logistics · Supplier selection · Stochastic programming

1 Introduction

Natural disaster like hurricanes, earthquakes, volcano eruptions, and others, represent great logistical challenges because of their unpredictability. Every time a catastrophic event occurs in a community, it leaves behind dozens of victims, damaged infrastructure, a polluted environment, and disruptions in services like water and electricity. Humanitarian organizations (among many other actors) make great efforts to coordinate the

J. A. Marmolejo-Saucedo et al. (Eds.): COMPSE 2020, LNICST 359, pp. 31–51, 2021.
https://doi.org/10.1007/978-3-030-69839-3_3

procurement of relief items; they recruit volunteers, perform search and rescue activities; they purchase machinery, or any item needed by the first responders, and many other plans are executed. If the procurement of these items is done after the disaster, humanitarian organizations may find scarce or overpriced products that make the procurement costs very high. Considering that many of these organizations do not sell products or make profits, it could be very difficult to fund the procurement of such items; indeed, they expect to receive donations from the community or have a budget allocated by the local government.

It is known that when a disaster or an emergency occurs, there are many people involved willing to help such as mass media, local and international governments, volunteers, Non-governmental organizations (NGO) and a long list of donors who form the humanitarian supply chain. However, the great number of people involved could make the logistics very complex and difficult. On top of that, the time plays an important role in humanitarian logistics since the victims need immediate assistance and cannot wait long for help. It becomes a matter of life and death.

One of the strategies that has been addressed regarding the post-disaster procurement is the pre-positioned inventory. Some organizations have the capability of storing large quantities of items as prevention when a disaster arises, nevertheless, as it may be expected, this strategy carries out large administrative and inventory costs. As explained before, some (or many) humanitarian organizations have limited funds and many do not have a warehouse to store items, tools and machinery, or the resources to hire personnel to administrate it. This is relevant due to the importance of considering the available budget of an organization.

In 2001, the International Federation of Red Cross and Red Crescent Society (IFRC) adopted Framework agreements as part of their strategy to procure humanitarian relief items. These agreements seek to reduce costs and delivery lead times when a disaster occurs. In a Framework Agreement, the supplier reserves an agreed capacity for the buyer who commits to purchase the number of items established in a given period of time (also called 'horizon'). The agreements are usually placed for standard items or high-volume items. This strategy turns out to be beneficial for both, suppliers and humanitarian organizations. On the one hand, the humanitarian organization, secures the supply of such items given and sudden-onset disaster; prior to settling the agreement, the organization is able to negotiate pricing according to the volume of purchase. On the other hand, the supplier is able to sell volume and could negotiate penalty fees in case of a breach between the reserved capacity and the actual purchase.

One important aspect of establishing contracts is the price negotiation that comes with it. Many suppliers offer price discounts depending of the volume of the purchase. This is beneficial for humanitarian organizations given their limited funds and the large volumes that are required for some items.

Some HO's that are directly linked to their local governments are given, by law, the responsibility to plan out strategies in order to assist during and after a disaster. These statutory agencies may receive annual funds that could be use in case of emergencies and the resource ought to be used wisely if the organization wants to fulfill the unpredicted demand.

We have to emphasize that at this point that the decision about what supplier the organization must procure from, already considers a set of suppliers approved to supply the products that are going to be needed in terms of quality, supplier coverage, price and quantity. This implicates that the organizations ought to run a previous assessment and advise the suppliers that were approved by the agency, nevertheless, the final decision will be made after the optimization presented in this work.

We address the supplier selection decision of a statutory agency with a limited budget but with the possibility of being assisted by the federal government; we propose a two-stage stochastic programming model given the nature of disasters and emergencies. The organization is willing to establish framework agreements with approved suppliers that are able to supply different relief items. Given the uncertainty of the demand, we build scenarios based on historical data from a specific region and denote the scenario formulation. The organization will commit to purchase the reserved capacity established in the agreement. However, we do not consider penalty costs given the fact that in the regional context of our case study, the government cannot be penalized by a civilian or a company for the breach of contract.

In Sect. 2 we address supplier selection tools and in Sect. 3 we do a general review of humanitarian logistics. In Sect. 4 a literature review is shown. Section 5 explains the methodology followed for this work. Section 6 explains the experimentation and the case instance. In Sect. 7 we comment on the results of the instance, and in Sect. 8 we make conclusions to this work.

2 Supplier Selection

Procurement refers to the different activities such as transportation, purchasing, tracking and traceability of the merchandise; supplier development and supplier selection. Procurement could translate in a great competitive advantage for an organization depending on the criteria chosen to carry out the supplier selection. This selection must be aligned to the objectives and strategies of the company as their performance also depends on their commercial partners [1].

The globalization has expanded the supply worldwide. Suppliers are located farther away making supply chains more complex and delivery lead times longer [2]. Thus, it is important to develop strategies that simplify the procurement of products through the appropriate selection of commercial partners that help ensure on-time deliveries and product availability [3].

Nevertheless, supplier selection is normally a complex activity given the qualitative criteria involved. Some authors have proposed multi-criteria tools as a first stage on the selection and optimization tools in a later stage.

The use of quantitative approaches has been broadly studied by different authors. [2] and [1] present state-of-the-art supplier selection tools that have been addressed. Throughout the purchasing process, they identify the pre-qualification methods that are useful to shorten the supplier base, and the final decision methods that help optimize the final purchase of items from an approved base of reliable suppliers.

Pre-qualification methods include and are not limited to:

- Categorical methods.
- Fuzzy set theory.
- Data envelopment analysis.
- Case-based reasoning.
- Analytical hierarchy process.

Final decision methods include and are not limited to:

- Linear and non-linear mathematical programming.
- Mixed integer programming.
- Meta-programming.
- Multi-objective programming.

In a competitive environment where multiple suppliers offer similar quality and performance, decisions are likely to be made based on pricing. In some cases, these decisions are based on quality or lead time, depending on the nature of the company.

Procurement from different sources occurs when a single supplier cannot meet the demand, thus, the buyer must allocate the demand to multiple suppliers.

Organizations also have to make decisions as to how many candidates will be part of their selected pool of suppliers. Allocating full demand to a single supplier could carry important risks of interruption of flow throughout the chain if any unpredicted event arises. On the other hand, having multiple sources may increase administration costs and establishing strong relationships becomes hard to manage. It is important for organizations to maintain a robust yet adequately small supplier base so that costs are kept low and performance remains high.

3 Humanitarian Logistics

Humanitarian logistics is defined as the process of planning, implementing and controlling the cost-efficient and effective flow and storing of goods and materials, and the related information, from the point of origin to the point of consumption to ease the suffering of vulnerable people [4, 5].

A disaster is an event that has great negative impact in the society and its environment. It could be natural-made such as hurricanes, earthquakes and volcanic eruptions; or man-made like air crashes, nuclear accidents or wars. Natural disasters, in particular, represent great logistical challenges due to the on-sudden event and the uncertainty that it holds.

In the last decades, through the opening of mass media, people all over the world has been aware of the catastrophic consequences of natural disasters on large and small populations, and the great economic impacts that they carry.

[4] identifies four stages in the humanitarian chains, two before and two after the disaster.

In the mitigation stage, the community runs risk assessments on infrastructure and roads, and if necessary, construction of systems to reduce the damage of a disaster like the anti-tsunami systems that Japan put in place.

In the preparedness stage, the community carries out activities such as the recruitment of volunteers, education of the society in regards of emergencies, acquisition of vehicles and emergency tools; storing of relief items and the development of emergency plans to be executed in case of a crisis.

After the disasters, the response stage is immediately triggered. Some of the activities in this stage include, search and rescue of people, data collection regarding the disaster zone, establishment of shelters, and transportation of humanitarian relief items.

Lastly, the rehabilitation stage begins usually weeks after de disaster and the activities performed in this stage target the re-establishment of normality within the community.

Many organizations use to procure the relief items after the disaster, also called post-disaster procurement. Nevertheless, due to the high demand of relief items, prices are usually expensive or and products are scarce. If the HO is able to procure these items, the delivery lead times are usually long which is not aligned to the objective of the humanitarian logistics. Some authors have proposed to keep a pre-positioned inventory [3, 6, 7], this is, to store relief items in the preparedness stage so that the humanitarian organization is able to start shipping to the affected zones immediately after a disaster strike. This, of course, would be ideal if humanitarian organizations had enough funds, staff, space and budget to keep a large warehouse operating. Unfortunately, this is not the case for most of HO's. Keeping pre-positioned inventory means high storing costs, complex administration and risk of obsolescence, since many of the relief items may be perishable. [6] have proposed the use of framework agreements. By settling an agreement or contract with commercial partners, the integration of the humanitarian chain becomes stronger, since terms such as pricing, quality, packaging and lead time are established before the actual purchase.

Humanitarian relief items are usually believed to be first-aid items like bottled water, food, or medicines. Nevertheless, items such as peak axes, shovels, gloves and other materials use to carry out the actual rescue activities during the response stage can also be considered as relief items. Depending on their objectives and internal administration, HO's may procure first-aid items or tools necessary for perform such activities.

3.1 Differences Between Commercial Logistics and Humanitarian Logistics

Commercial logistics have been broadly studied. The main objective is to maximize the profit of products, services and information moved along the supply chain. Although, humanitarian logistics move, not only products, but also people, the main objective is to ease the suffering of vulnerable people.

Whereas in commercial chain, we speak about a relatively stable demand, humanitarian logistics stands before a very irregular and unexpected demand; the time, place or quantity remain unknown but until the disaster has ocurred. Some authors have developed scenario-based stochastic programming models to normalize demand. This is, they collect information from past events to somehow determine patterns, means, and statistics to structure possible scenarios [6, 8].

Another great difference is the people that are involved. Common parties in commercial chains are suppliers and/or service providers, distributors, warehouses, third-party logistics, customs, and others; an interdependency along the chain exists and all parties seek to maximize their benefits and be effective and cost-efficient. In humanitarian logistics we observe parties like donors, HO's, churches, governments, volunteers, warehouses, suppliers, transportation providers, among others, seeking to bring help all at the same time (many of these with their own agendas and interests); some of these parties even take advantage of the mass media to advertise their products as a marketing strategy. At the same time, even the local citizens, toss away unnecessary items that they no longer need.

Commercial logistics have a broad performance validation based on international standards of the supply chain. A clear example of this is the six-sigma methodology, the SCORE model, and others. In the humanitarian fields, a performance indicator is usually the response time, fill rate, percentage of demand satisfied and the expectations of donors [9]. See Table 1.

Table 1. Differences between commercial logistics and humanitarian logistics.

	Commercial logistics	Humanitarian logistics
Objective	Maximize profit	Save lives and ease suffering
Demand	Generally stable	Irregular
Human resources	Professional careers	High rotation of volunteers
Resource flow	Commercial products	People, food, shelter, etc.
Stakeholder	Shareholders, customers	Donors, governments, NGO's, etc.
Inventory control	Safety stocks in place	Difficult to control
Performance validation	Standard to the supply chain	Response time, % of demand covered

4   Literature Review

Supplier selection has a large list of scientific and academic papers. For this literature review, we used: "supplier selection", "supplier evaluation", and "humanitarian logistics". In the most recent papers from the last five years from the National Consortium for Scientific and Technological Information Resources (CONRICYT) data base, we find the ones from [3] and [10] who develop a two-stage stochastic programming model to analyze the pre-positioned inventory at the supplier's expense. [11] propose a stochastic programming model to resolve the optimal stock quantity reducing costs of transportation, penalty and inventory; similarly, [12] integrate carrier and supplier selection for developing contractual agreements, they use a scenario-based two-stage stochastic programming model for the establishment of joint decision-making and help minimize the fixed contract costs, commodity and vehicle reservation costs, commodity purchasing costs, vehicle rental costs, transportation costs, and others. The work of [13] proposes a bi-objective mixed possibilistic, two-stage stochastic programming model to strengthen the decision-making process considering risks of disruptions in the chain as well as the suppliers profiles based on the action plans in case of a major disruption. [14] propose a multi-stage programming model to minimize the expected costs of having an agreement in place and procuring relief items from the suppliers. They consider commitment quantities of the relief agency, reserve capacity of suppliers, and discount rates. [6] considers framework agreements with suppliers establishing a fixed agreement fee and reserved capacity. [8] also propose a two-stage stochastic programming model based in scenarios and then compare it with a chance-constrained programming (CCP) model that assumes a probability distribution and restricts the probability of not covering the demand. Despite the work of [15] and [16] is not in humanitarian logistics, they use the analytics hierarchy process (AHP) and the technique for order of preference by similarity to ideal solution (TOPSIS) respectively, to later combine it with Mixed Integer Programming (MIP) by inserting the data obtained from the previous methods in order to optimize it. [17] develop a supply partner framework for continuous-aid procurement using fuzzy AHP and fuzzy TOPSIS to rank different supplier alternatives. They identify 6 attributes and 24 sub-criteria that consider relevant for the multi-criteria decision-making problem.

[18] use a multi-criteria decision-making tool, TOPSIS, to help on the supplier selection problem for the blood-bag industry and take into consideration attributes such as product quality, delivery performance, financial status, purchasing costs, personnel and facilities.

We have identified that literature in humanitarian logistics is not as extensive as in commercial chains, nevertheless, we have found important works on the field. Stochastic programming is the tool found in most works for supplier selection.

We see that only the work of [16] considered a budget despite it is an important factor for many HO given the limited funds. We believe that it's important to address budget constraints in the humanitarian field for the final decision methods that have been previously addressed by other authors (Table 2).

Table 2. Literature review.

	Humanitarian Logistics	Supplier Selection	Item procurement	Budget	Pre-positioned inventory	Solution	Tool
[10]	x	x	x		x	Optimal	Stochastic programming
[3]	x	x	x		x	Optimal	Stochastic programming
[11]	x	x	x		x	Optimal	Stochastic programming
[13]	x	x	x		x	Optimal	Stochastic programming
[6]	x	x	x			Optimal	Stochastic programming
[8]		x	x			Optimal	Stochastic programming/CCP
[15]		x	x			Approximate	AHP/MIP

(*continued*)

Table 2. (*continued*)

	Humanitarian Logistics	Supplier Selection	Item procurement	Budget	Pre-positioned inventory	Solution	Tool
[16]		x	x	x		Optimal	Fuzzy TOPSIS/MIP
[12]	x	x	x			Optimal	Stochastic programming
[14]	x	x	x		x	Optimal	Stochastic programming
[17]	x	x				Approximate	Fuzzy AHP and fuzzy TOPSIS
[18]		x	x			Approximate	TOPSIS

5   Methodology

Given the literature review, we have followed the methodology proposed in [19] for the formulation of mathematical models:

1. Formulate the problem.
2. Observe the system.
3. Formulate a mathematical problem for the problem.
4. Verify the model.
5. Select a suitable alternative.

5.1   Problem Description

A statutory agency seeks to make decisions as to what suppliers must they purchase from when a sudden-onset disaster occurs. The organization receives an annual budget from the federal government that is available for emergencies only. For 2020 the budget was $21 million pesos. The organization procures first need items and machinery through the Procurement Office. These purchases are made in different ways; however, it is known that tender processes can be done and that the organization can establish framework agreements with suppliers.

A list of suppliers already approved by the organization exists, however, there are many suppliers that are candidates to use. Only the suppliers in the list can be selected in case of an emergency. The suppliers may have different characteristics and offer different deals. The reserved capacity, the unit price and the coverage may differ from one another.

Another important information is that in case of a high-impact disaster that exceeds the capacity of the organization to help the population, the organization can procure the items needs from the federal government. The procurement of this items is not monetary which means that the organizations has specific quantities to request to the federation.

The suppliers offer discounts depending on the volume of the purchase. The price will also depend on the shipping destination and the requested lead time. The suppliers may offer different pricing schedule for each region depending on their coverage. We assume that these prices will always be better or lower enough to buying the items in the spot market (post-disaster procurement).

The organization has to define the minimum and maximum number of suppliers to be selected. It is important to pinpoint that the more suppliers available for selection, the higher the costs of procuring. On the other hand, if the organization was to pick only one supplier, there is a high risk of falling short on demand coverage if a medium or high-impact disaster occurs.

5.2 Regional Context

For the case study we take the Mexican state of Nuevo Leon. It holds a population of 5.13 million habitants and 80% inhabit the metropolitan area. Historically, the state has been impacted every year for severe storms and hurricanes. Between 2000 and 2015, eleven storms were categorized as natural disaster. In more recent years, the storm "Fernand" in 2019 and "Hanna" in 2020 were also categorized as natural disasters.

Storms that form in the Atlantic Ocean are common to pass through the Gulf of Mexico and hit the Mexican coasts every year. Studies ran by several government institutions determine that Nuevo Leon is likely to be struck by Tropical Storms, and Hurricanes categories II and III in the scale of Saffir-Simpson. See Table 3.

Table 3. Saffir-Simpson hurricane wind scale.

Category	Winds	Damages
I	119–153 km/h	Minimum damage
II	154–177 km/h	Moderate damage
III	178–208 km/h	Important damage
IV	209–251 km/h	Severe damage
V	Above 252 km/h	Catastrophic damage

The State capital, Monterrey, is the third largest city in Mexico and given the fact that it holds eighty percent of the population, storms cause great damages to the population and the infrastructure of the city and its metropolitan area. Annually, the state accumulates 650 mm with rains that are mostly seen in the summer.

5.3 Model Formulation

We use the following notation for the supplier selection problem:

Sets	
I:	Set of candidate suppliers
K:	Set of items
L:	Set of delivery lead time intervals
M:	Set of quantity intervals offered by supplier i for item k
R:	Set of demand regions
S:	Set of scenarios
Parameters	
p_s:	Probability of scenario s
η_{min}:	Minimum number of suppliers to select
η_{max}:	Maximum number of suppliers to select
d_{kr}^s:	Demand of product k for region in scenario s
z_{kl}^s:	Portion of demand to be satisfied in interval l for product k in scenario s
v_{ik}^{max}:	Maximum capacity reserved for item k from supplier i
f_i:	Fixed agreement costs supplier i
α_{iklmr}^s:	Lower breakpoint associated with quantity interval m offered by supplier i, for item k, serving region r, within the lead time interval l in scenario s
β_{iklmr}^s:	Upper breakpoint associated with quantity interval m offered by supplier I, for item k, serving region r, within the lead time interval l in scenario s
u_{iklmr}:	Unit price offered by supplier i for delivering purchased item k at quantity interval m, to serve region r, within the lead time interval l, in scenario s
ω_{kr}:	Unit price offered by the external source at quantity interval m, to serve region r, within the lead time interval l, in scenario s
Ψ:	Budget allocated by the agency for the procurement of k
Variables	
Q_{iklmr}^s:	Amount purchased of item k from supplier i at quantity interval m, to serve region r, within the lead time interval l, in scenario s
E_{kr}^s:	Amount purchased of item k from the external source at quantity interval m, to serve region r, within the lead time interval l, in scenario s
$Y_i =$	1, if the supplier i is selected for the agreement; 0, otherwise
$X_{iklmr}^s =$	1, if the agreement with supplier i is executed by purchasing item k at quantity interval m, to serve region r, within the lead time interval l in scenario s

The problem is formulated as follows:

$$\min \sum_{i \in I} \sum_{k \in K} f_i Y_i$$

$$+ \sum_{s \in S} p_s \left[\sum_{i \in I} \sum_{k \in K} \sum_{l \in L} \sum_{m \in M} \sum_{r \in R} u_{iklmr} Q^s_{kilmr} + \sum_{k \in K} \sum_{r \in R} \omega_{iklmr} E^s_{kr} \right] \tag{1}$$

Subject to:

$$\sum_{i \in I} \sum_{k \in K} Y_{ik} \geq \eta_{min} \qquad \forall i \in I \tag{2}$$

$$\sum_{i \in I} \sum_{k \in K} Y_{ik} \leq \eta_{máx} \qquad \forall i \in I \tag{3}$$

$$\sum_{i \in I} \sum_{l \in L} \sum_{m \in M} Q^s_{iklmr} + E^s_{kr} \geq d^s_{kr} \qquad \forall k \in K, r \in R, s \in S \tag{4}$$

$$\sum_{i \in I} \sum_{l \in L} \sum_{m \in M} \sum_{r \in R} Q^s_{iklmr} \geq d^s_{kr} 10\% \qquad \forall k \in K, s \in S \tag{5}$$

$$\sum_{l \in L} \sum_{m \in M} Q^s_{kilmr} \leq v^{máx}_{ik} Y_{ik} \qquad \forall i \in I, k \in K, r \in R, s \in S \tag{6}$$

$$\sum_{i \in I} \sum_{m \in M} Q^s_{iklmr} \geq z^s_{kl} d^s_{kr} \qquad \forall i \in I, k \in K, l \in L, r \in R, s \in S \tag{7}$$

$$Q^s_{kilmr} \geq X^s_{kilmr} \alpha_{iklmr} \qquad \forall i \in I, k \in K, l \in L, m \in M, r \in R, s \in S \tag{8}$$

$$Q^s_{kilmr} \geq X^s_{kilmr} \beta_{iklmr} \qquad \forall i \in I, k \in K, l \in L, m \in M, r \in R, s \in S \tag{9}$$

$$\sum_{m \in M} X^s_{kilmr} \leq Y_i \qquad \forall i \in I, k \in K, l \in L, r \in R, s \in S \tag{10}$$

$$\sum_{i \in I} \sum_{k \in K} \sum_{l \in L} \sum_{m \in M} \sum_{r \in R} u_{iklmr} Q^s_{iklmr} + \sum_{i \in I} f_i Y_i \leq \Psi \tag{11}$$

$$Q^s_{iklmr} \in \mathbb{Z}^+_0 \qquad \forall i \in I, k \in K, l \in L, m \in M, r \in R, s \in S \tag{12}$$

$$E^s_{kr} \in \mathbb{Z}^+_0 \qquad \forall k \in K, r \in R, s \in S \tag{13}$$

$$X^s_{iklmr} \in \{1, 0\} \qquad \forall i \in I, k \in K, l \in L, m \in M, r \in R, s \in S \tag{14}$$

$$Y_i \in \{1, 0\} \qquad \forall i \in I \tag{15}$$

Where the objective function (1) seeks to reduce procurement and agreement costs. In a first stage, it makes the decision as to what suppliers are selected; in stage two, it reduces the procurement costs associated to those suppliers and the procurement from a higher-level source (federal government). Constraint (2) and (3) are the minimum and maximum number of candidate suppliers to use. (4) ensures that the demand is covered by sourcing from the selected suppliers and from the higher-level source. (5) ensures that at least 10% of the demand is covered by the suppliers for each item. (6) ensures that the reserved capacity is not exceeded. (7) indicates the level of service, which indicates the portion of the demand to be satisfied in a determined delivery lead time interval. (8) and (9) ensure that the items are procured within the lead time and quantity intervals. (10) ensures that the items are only procured from the selected suppliers. (11) is the budget constraint. (12) and (13) are the integer variables, and (14) and (15) are binary variables.

6 Experimentation

6.1 Scenario Formulation

The parameter p_s of the mathematical model represents the probability of occurrence of a determined scenario. To formulate the scenarios, we have looked into the possible development of a disaster in the region. Particularly, this region is hit by tropical storms, and hurricanes categories II and III, which are considered to be low, medium and high impact phenomena respectively. These commonly land by the coast of the Gulf of Mexico and make their path to the state of Nuevo Leon.

The State evaluates the risk in the territory and divide it in 5 regions: north, south, west, citrus, and metro. Specifically, the citrus and west regions are considered to be always hit by these phenomena due to their geographical position and given the track of hydrometeorological disasters.

By making possible combinations of regions affected, we identify six possible combinations shown in Table 4.

Table 4. Combination of affected regions.

Combination	Fixed regions	Region
1	Citrus – West	North
2		South
3		Metro
4		Metro – North
5		Metro – South
6		Metro – North – South

We discard the combination where regions are impacted except the metro region (Citrus–West–North–South) as we believe it is very unlikely that a storm affects both, the north and the south regions but not the metro that is located between these two.

6.2 Probability of Occurrence

For each disaster impact we would consider each of the six combinations given before, which makes a total of 18 possible scenarios. The sum of the probability of occurrence must be equal to 1, this is $\sum_{s \in S} p_s = 1$. For that, we estimate it as follows:

1. A random number is generated for each scenario, $\bar{p}_s$. Depending on the disaster impact a random number with normal distribution is generated, U[80,100], U[20,40], and U[0,20] for tropical storms, hurricane category II and hurricane category III, respectively.
2. Each number $\bar{p}_s$ is divided by the sum of all random numbers. $p_s = \bar{p}_s / \sum_{s \in S} \bar{p}_s$.

The tree of scenarios can be observed in Fig. 1 where the 18 scenarios are shown and their probability of occurrence which was estimated using the steps described above. We observe that the probability of occurrence in scenarios where the regions are affected by tropical storms have a higher probability than those scenarios where hurricanes category III strike.

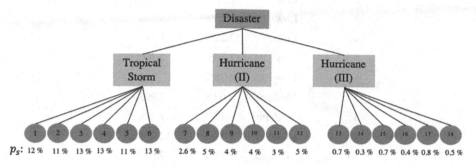

p_s: 12%   11%   13%   13%   11%   13%   2.6% 5%   4%   4%   3%   5%   0.7% 0.3% 0.7% 0.4% 0.8% 0.5%

Fig. 1. Tree of scenarios – probability of occurrence

6.3 Demand Scenarios

For each disaster impact we generate a possible demand which represents the number of people affected by the storm. The demand will be low, medium and high for tropical storms, hurricanes category II and hurricanes category III respectively. The unit of measure for items k will be calculated based on the result of this demand. We followed the steps below to calculate demand:

1. We generate a random number with uniform distribution for each region that is affected in a determined scenario with exemption of those that are not.
2. We multiply the demand by the percentage of population concentrated in that region. North, west, south and citrus hold 5%, and the metro region holds 80% of the population.
3. We obtain the total demand per scenario.

The minimum and maximum of victims in point 1 is to be determined based on historical data for the region of case study. According to the history of Nuevo León, we generate numbers as follows: 100 – 5,000 victims in case of tropical storms; 5,000 – 15,000 in case of hurricane category II; and 15,000 – 50,000 in case of hurricane category III. The total victims per scenario is shown in Table 5.

Table 5. Number of victims per scenario.

Scenario#	Impact	Probability	Total victims
1	Low	12.48%	501
2	Low	12.75%	183
3	Low	11.83%	3,556
4	Low	12.22%	2,812
5	Low	12.75%	2,300
6	Low	10.78%	994
7	Medium	2.63%	1,993
8	Medium	3.15%	1,318
9	Medium	5.12%	12,974
10	Medium	5.12%	7,578
11	Medium	3.55%	10,275
12	Medium	3.55%	6,555
13	High	0.26%	4,727
14	High	0.13%	4,683
15	High	1.31%	33,427
16	High	0.26%	37,239
17	High	1.18%	20,218
18	High	0.92%	38,782

6.4 Case Instance

For the experimentation, we considered two items: bottled water and blankets.

Water is vital for humans. For the demand generation of bottled water, we estimated a 2 L consumption per person per seven days. This means that each victim will require 14 L of water. The standard presentation of bottled water is a 24 pack of bottles of 500 ml, or packs with 12 L.

Blankets are required by victims that had to be reallocated to a community shelter. For the case instance, we considered that only 30% of the victims require shelter, thus, they will need a blanket. No further specifications for blankets were considered.

The demand of each items is presented in Table 6, where the demand for water was calculated multiplying the total victims in each scenario by 14, and by 0.30 for blankets.

We also consider a supplier base of 10 candidates, 5 for each item and a fixed cost for singing an agreement with any of the candidates. The cost is $1,000.

Table 6. Demand scenarios per item.

Scenario#	Scaled Prob.	Bottled water					Blankets				
		West	Citrus	North	South	Metro	West	Citrus	North	South	Metro
1	12.48%	275	46	264	0	0	71	12	68	0	0
2	12.75%	17	85	0	112	0	4	22	0	29	0
3	11.83%	127	108	0	0	3914	33	28	0	0	1007
4	12.22%	281	257	187	0	2555	72	66	48	0	657
5	12.75%	35	153	0	157	2337	9	39	0	40	601
6	10.78%	117	243	121	153	525	30	62	31	39	135
7	2.63%	822	728	776	0	0	211	187	200	0	0
8	3.15%	337	772	0	429	0	87	198	0	110	0
9	5.12%	408	855	0	0	13874	105	220	0	0	3568
10	5.12%	480	468	781	0	7112	123	120	201	0	1829
11	3.55%	318	386	0	621	10662	82	99	0	160	2742
12	3.55%	617	406	808	506	5310	159	104	208	130	1365
13	0.26%	2849	175	891	0	0	733	456	229	0	0
14	0.13%	2067	196	0	1460	0	532	498	0	375	0
15	1.31%	2746	1187	0	0	35064	706	305	0	0	9017
16	0.26%	1117	1302	2519	0	38507	287	335	648	0	9902
17	1.18%	1313	2783	0	1084	18408	338	716	0	279	4734
18	0.92%	1701	1500	2733	2402	36910	437	386	703	618	9491

The minimum purchase of each item is 100 units. Nevertheless, suppliers offer a 5% discount in purchases over 1,000 units of bottled water, or 500 blankets. Prices, and quantity and lead time intervals are shown in Table 7.

As per the costs of procuring from the federal government ($\omega_{kr}E_{kr}^s$) we establish a price large enough to not be selected as a first choice but until the reserved capacity or the budget is used up.

It is also assumed that the agency established the first lead time interval to be from 5–7 days, and the second lead time to be 8–10 days; and wishes a to supply at least 30% of the demand within the first lead time interval. This means that the selected candidate suppliers must deliver the item(s) within 5 to 7 days. Lastly, the agency holds an annual budget of 21 million pesos for 2020. We assume that the agency wishes to allocate 1.5 million to the procurement of these two items. According to the formulated mathematical model, the associated costs to the procurement of bottled water and blanked must not exceed the assigned budget.

This model was run using the General Algebraic Modeling System (GAMS) using the solver CPLEX. An equipment with processor AMD A6–3620 APU 2.20 GHz and 6 GB RAM was used.

Table 7. Prices offered by suppliers.

	Supplier	Price < 100 units	Price within 2nd quantity interval	Price within 2nd delivery lead time interval
Bottled water	1	$ 81.00	$ 76.95	$ 73.10
	2	$ 90.00	$ 85.50	$ 81.23
	3	$ 93.00	$ 88.35	$ 83.93
	4	$ 80.00	$ 75.00	$ 72.20
	5	$ 83.00	$ 78.85	$ 74.91
Blankets	6	$ 133.00	$ 126.35	$ 120.03
	7	$ 129.00	$ 122.55	$ 116.42
	8	$ 120.00	$ 144.00	$ 108.30
	9	$ 135.00	$ 128.25	$ 121.84
	10	$ 122.00	$ 115.90	$ 110.11

7 Results

The instance was solved in 0.171 min for 14,591 variables and the results are presented in Table 8.

Table 8. Results.

	Results
Selected suppliers	3
Suppliers of bottled water	2
Suppliers of blankets	1
Procurement costs (thousands)	$ 1,496.95
Fixed costs (thousands)	$ 3.00
Total costs (thousands)	$ 1,499.95
Demand satisfied by selected suppliers	56%
Demand satisfied by the federal government	44%

Observation 1. From the 10-supplier base, only 3 candidates were selected, two suppliers of water bottled and 1 of supplier of blankets. Given the prices listed on Table 6, the results show to be aligned as the selected candidates were the ones with the lower price offer.

Observation 2. The budget is used up at 100% without surpassing it. This indicates that the budget constraint has been honored in the execution. With this solution we can cover up 100% of the demand in scenarios from 1 to 14; and up until 56% in for the rest. The uncovered demand must be covered by the federal government.

Observation 3. It is observed that the relief items to procure in the first lead time interval is 60% for bottled water and 76% for blankets which indicate that the service level of 30% at the first lead time interval was honored.

Observation 4. We observe a small surplus of 0.48%. This is due to the minimum purchases established by the suppliers that had to be procured even when the demand was lower than the minimum, mostly in the scenarios under tropical storms.

7.1 Budget Analysis

Observation 5. We adjusted the budget parameter to see the performance and the behavior of our model. If the parameter Ψ is set under 1.5 million pesos, the stochastic model will be infeasible, as it is not possible to meet the demand of at least 10% indicated in constraint 5. Nevertheless, by increasing the budget, the agency is able to select even more suppliers and satisfy the demand. By reaching up to 4.75 million pesos in budget, the agency is able to satisfy the demand with the allocated resource without going through the process of sourcing from the federal government. See Table 9.

Table 9. Budget allocation analysis.

Budget ($)	Suppliers selected	Request aid from federal government?
Less than 1.5 million	Infeasible	Yes
1.5 million	3	Yes
2 million	4	Yes
2.5 million	5	Yes
2.75 million	5	Yes
3 million	6	Yes
4 million	7	Yes
4.75 million	7	No

As mentioned above, monetary resources are very important for HO's. This brief analysis could be of help to a statutory agency in the decision-making process as to how much budget must be allocated for certain relief items or tooling. At the same time, it helps the agency to understand the range of minimum and maximum budget allocation; on the one hand it is important to cover at least 10% of the demand generated for bottled water and blankets, nevertheless, it would not be possible by allocating Less than 1.5 million pesos. On the other hand, the agency could make a decision as to how much more resources allocate to these relief items; by allocating the maximum budget, 4.75 million, the state government would not be in need to request aid from the federal government and would meet the demand from their own resources, saving time and of course, lives, since it may take more waiting time to transport federal resources to the disaster zone.

7.2 Deterministic Solutions

The GAMS code of the presented model was built in such fashion that it also provides deterministic solutions for each scenario taking the random demand as a known parameter. In this way, we are able to compare the solution provided by the stochastic model versus eighteen solutions of the deterministic version of the model. We can observe the results in Tables 9, 10 and 11.

Table 10. Deterministic solutions I.

		Deterministic model (tropical storm)					
	Stochastic model	S1	S2	S3	S4	S5	S6
Candidate suppliers selected	3	3	2	2	2	2	2
Bottled water	2	2	1	1	1	1	1
Blankets	1	1	1	1	1	1	1
Procurement costs (thousands)	$1,496.95	$87.12	$60.96	$441.77	$357.17	$309.85	$156.92
Fixed costs (thousands)	$3.00	$3.00	$2.00	$2.00	$2.00	$2.00	$2.00
Total (thousands)	$1,499.95	$90.12	$62.96	$443.77	$359.17	$311.85	$158.92
Budget used	100%	6%	4%	30%	24%	21%	11%

Table 11. Deterministic solutions II.

		Deterministic model (hurricane category II)					
	Stochastic model	S7	S8	S9	S10	S11	S12
Candidate suppliers selected	3	2	2	3	2	3	2
Bottled water	2	1	1	2	1	2	1
Blankets	1	1	1	1	1	1	1
Procurement costs (thousands)	$1,496.95	$257.84	$172.00	$149.70	$914.41	$1,233.70	$799.20
Fixed costs (thousands)	$3.00	$2.00	$2.00	$3.00	$2.00	$3.00	$2.00
Total (thousands)	$1,499.95	$259.84	$174.00	$152.70	$916.41	$1,236.70	$801.20
Budget used	100%	17%	12%	10%	61%	82%	53%

Observation 6. We observe that the organization can satisfy the demand with 1.5 million pesos in 80% of the scenarios. This is important for decision-making as to how much budget to allocate and what suppliers are the best candidates (Table 12).

Table 12. Deterministic solutions III.

| | Stochastic model | Deterministic model (hurricane category III) | | | | | |
		S13	S14	S15	S16	S17	S18
Candidate suppliers selected	3	2	2	3	3	3	3
Bottled water	2	1	1	2	2	2	2
Blankets	1	1	1	1	1	1	1
Procurement costs (thousands)	$1,496.95	$577.25	$568.94	$1,496.67	$1,496.99	$1,496.97	$1,496.95
Fixed costs (thousands)	$3.00	$2.00	$2.00	$3.00	$3.00	$3.00	$3.00
Total (thousands)	$1,499.95	$579.25	$570.94	$1,499.67	$1,499.99	$1,499.97	$1,499.95
Budget used	100%	39%	38%	100%	100%	100%	100%

After the observations previously made, we determine that the model delivers a logical solution. It is important to keep in mind that the procurement costs are those of $u_{iklmr}Q^s_{iklmr}$, and that the costs of E^s_{kr}, are auxiliary costs for the mathematical compilation purpose. Binary variables X^s_{iklmr} and Y_i are also coherent to the solution delivered for Q^s_{iklmr}, this is, the contracts and the suppliers that are selected correspond to the suppliers to procure the items from.

8   Conclusions

Humanitarian logistics are of special attention for many societies. Its main importance relies on the ease of suffering caused by natural (or man-made) disasters that have happened and will, probably, continue to happen.

Logistics per se, is a detailed plan which in humanitarian logistics takes place in the preparedness stage. HO's and the actors involved in humanitarian chains are able to improve their performance significantly through the planning and development of strategies that will be implemented in any of the stages of humanitarian logistics.

Given the important differences between commercial and humanitarian chains it's important to bring different approaches to help communities be better prepared for a humanitarian crisis.

This work seeks to help integrate the humanitarian chain by strengthening the relationships between suppliers and HO's by establishing framework agreements.

This research provides a quantitative approach for decision-making in humanitarian logistics. Results indicate that it is possible to minimize the costs associated to the procurement of humanitarian relief items by using stochastic programming as a supplier selections tool. Despite the use of mathematical programming in other papers, the main contribution of this work is based on the budget constraint given the limited funds of many humanitarian organizations and the possibility of estimating the procurement amounts of a higher-level source like the federal government in our case study. The model is able to provide information useful for the decision-making process within a humanitarian organization regarding budget allocation. The proposed model shows an optimal solution given the type of scenarios and its distribution of probability delivering a 100% of demand satisfied in fourteen scenarios and up to 58% of demand satisfied in scenarios where the it spikes considerably as a consequence of an important natural phenomenon.

The proposed model is not limited to the type of items nor to the type of disasters so we believed this could be adapted to different HO's that hold a limited budget.

References

1. Castro, S., et al.: Selección de proveedores: una aproximación al estado del arte. Cuad. Adm. **22**(38), 145–167 (2009)
2. De Boer, L., Labro, E., Morlacchi, P.: A review of methods supporting supplier selection. Eur. J. Purch. Supply Manag. **7**, 75–89 (2001)
3. Hu, S., Dong, Z.S.: Supplier selection and pre-positioning strategy in humanitarian relief. Omega **83**, 287–298 (2019)
4. Van Wassenhove, L.N.: Blackett memorial lecture humanitarian aid logistics: supply chain management in high gear. J. Oper. Res. Soc. **57**(5), 475–489 (2006)
5. Overstreet, R., Hall, D., Hanna, J., Kelly Rainer, R.: Research in humanitarian logistics. J. Humanit. Logist. Supply Chain Manag. **1**(2), 114–131 (2011). https://doi.org/10.1108/204 26741111158421
6. Balcik, B., Ak, D.: Supplier selection for framework agreements in humanitarian relief. Prod. Oper. Manag. **23**(6), 1028–1041 (2014)
7. Kunz, N., Reiner, G., Gold, S.: Investing in disaster management capabilities versus pre-positioning inventory: a new approach to disaster preparedness. Int. J. Prod. Econ. **157**, 261–272 (2014)
8. Li, L., Zabinsky, Z.B.: Incorporating uncertainty into a supplier selection problem. Int. J. Prod. Econ. **134**(2), 344–356 (2011)
9. Ertem, M.A., Buyurgan, N., Rossetti, M.D.: Multiple-buyer procurement auctions framework for humanitarian supply chain management. Int. J. Phys. Distrib. Logist. Manag. **40**(3), 202–227 (2010)
10. Aghajani, M., Torabi, S.A., Heydari, J.: A novel option contract integrated with supplier selection and inventory prepositioning for humanitarian relief supply chains. Socioecon. Plann. Sci. **71**, 100780 (2020)
11. Hu, S.L., Han, C.F., Meng, L.P.: Stochastic optimization for joint decision making of inventory and procurement in humanitarian relief. Comput. Ind. Eng. **111**, 39–49 (2017)
12. Ghorbani, M., Ramezanian, R.: Integration of carrier selection and supplier selection problem in humanitarian logistics. Comput. Ind. Eng. **144**, 106473 (2020)

13. Torabi, S.A., Baghersad, M., Mansouri, S.A.: Resilient supplier selection and order allocation under operational and disruption risks. Transp. Res. Part E Logist. Transp. Rev. **79**, 22–48 (2015)
14. Olanrewaju, O.G., Dong, Z.S., Hu, S.: Supplier selection decision making in disaster response. Comput. Ind. Eng. **143**, 106412 (2020)
15. Kisly, D., Tereso, A., Carvalho, M.S.: Implementation of multiple criteria decision analysis approaches in the supplier selection process: a case study. In: Rocha, Á., Correia, A., Adeli, H., Reis, L., Teixeira, M. (eds.) New Advances in Information Systems and Technologies. Advances in Intelligent Systems and Computing, vol. 444, pp. 951–960. Springer, Cham (2016). https://doi.org/10.1007/978-3-319-31232-3_90
16. Sahay, B.S., Gupta, S., Vinod Chandra Menon, N.: Managing humanitarian logistics (2015)
17. Venkatesh, V.G., Zhang, A., Deakins, E., Luthra, S., Mangla, S.: A fuzzy AHP-TOPSIS approach to supply partner selection in continuous aid humanitarian supply chains. Ann. Oper. Res. **283**(1–2), 1517–1550 (2018). https://doi.org/10.1007/s10479-018-2981-1
18. Venkatesh, V.G., Dubey, R., Joy, P., Thomas, M., Vijeesh, V., Moosa, A.: Supplier selection in blood bags manufacturing industry using TOPSIS model. Int. J. Oper. Res. **24**(4), 461–488 (2015)
19. Ziegel, E.R., Winston, W.: Operations research: applications and algorithms. Technometrics **30**(3), 361 (1988)

Image Classification Applied to the Detection of Leather Defects for Smart Manufacturing

Alberto Ochoa-Zezatti[1], Oliverio Cruz-Mejía[2(✉)], Jose Mejia[1],
and Hazael Ceron-Monroy[3]

[1] Universidad Autónoma de Ciudad Juárez, Ciudad Juárez, México
{alberto.ochoa,jose.mejia}@uacj.mx
[2] Universidad Autónoma del Estado de México, Toluca, México
ocruzm@uaemex.mx
[3] Universidad Anáhuac México, México City, México
hazael.ceron@anahuac.mx

Abstract. In the shoe production workshops, animal leather is used as the main raw material. Generally, an operator manually checks the surface of the leather, making sure that it does not present defects that compromise the quality of the final product.

This type of inspection is subject to human error and uncontrollable factors, which represents an opportunity for the automation of the process through a system of artificial vision.

A data set was developed consisting of images of animal leather, in good coordination and with defects.

The digitized samples were subjected to image processing using OpenCV and Scikit-Learn, and then used in a convolutional neural network interfacing, using TensorFlow's Keras library in Python.

Finally, the trained model is capable of classifying new images into two possible groups: "Defective Leather" and "Defect-free Leather".

The trained model offers 80% predictive accuracy and 85% reliability. Although the result can be considered satisfactory, it is expected to raise the mentioned percentage with a more robust data set than the one used for the project.

Keywords: Image classification · Artificial vision · Convolutional neural network · Smart manufacturing · Footwear industry · Keras · Tensorflow

1 Introduction

The Mexican footwear production industry has faced different challenges in recent years, derived from the competitiveness that has resulted from the opening of borders and the introduction of manufactured products in countries with the necessary resources to produce greater volumes with reduced production costs [1]. Therefore the need to develop and implement technologies focused on the optimization and automation of processes arises, which pose a better competitive scenario for Mexican companies.

© ICST Institute for Computer Sciences, Social Informatics and Telecommunications Engineering 2021
Published by Springer Nature Switzerland AG 2021. All Rights Reserved
J. A. Marmolejo-Saucedo et al. (Eds.): COMPSE 2020, LNICST 359, pp. 52–61, 2021.
https://doi.org/10.1007/978-3-030-69839-3_4

The relevance of this industry in Mexico is undeniable, since it represents 1.7% of the total manufacturing industries, contributing 2.4% of the total employment in this area. Likewise, the municipality of Leon, Guanajuato contributes with 57.8% of the total production value, being the municipality with the greatest participation. This makes it an ideal candidate for the application of technology-based projects focused on process optimization [2].

It is equally important to define the global situation of Mexico in footwear production, since in 2019 it reached the ninth place in the list of main producers, with a contribution of 268 million pairs during this year. The list is headed by China, with a contribution of 13,478 million pairs in the same period of time, according to the portal Statista [3].

In a shoe production workshop, animal leather is the main raw material. The quality of the final product is directly related to the quality of the leather used. This is susceptible to present diverse defects in its surface, among which we can find fissures, wrinles, scars and holes.

These defects will cause important quality failures in the final product, so it will be necessary to reprocess the product or directly discard it.

Defects are easily detected with proper lighting and training. Inspection of the leather surface is commonly performed by an operator, who checks and validates the condition of the material. Operator involvement adds complications related to low productivity, fatigue and subjectivity to the procedure [4].

It is possible to automate the inspection process by using an artificial vision system [5] that consists of processing and classifying images of animal leather, determining whether they have surface defects. For this purpose, it is necessary to develop an image classification system based on neuronal networks, which have been used before for the detection of defects in several areas, such as in the 3D impregnation process [6], in the automotive sector [7], in the agro-food industry [8] and, like this work, in the footwear industry [9].

Throughout this paper we present the process carried out for an image processing and classification system whose objective is to detect superficial defects in the leather used in the production of footwear and which can be easily integrated into an automated artificial vision system that informs by means of an alarm when anomalies are found.

1.1 Objective

Train a convolutional neural network which is capable of classifying an image (photoraph) of the leather surface into two possible categories: "with defects" or "without defects.

2 Fundamentals

Image classification based on neural networks has proven to be a powerful tool in the area of quality control, allowing an artificial vision system to be able to distinguish defective pieces, automating the inspection process with positive results in the area of footwear, specifically in animal leather [9, 10].

For an image classification system, it is convenient to train a convolutional neural network. These are a type of neuronal network that works with two-dimensional matrices, so it is frequently applied in the area of artificial vision [11]. In Fig. 1, it is illustrated the operation of such a network.

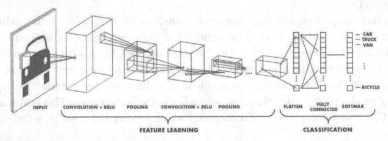

Fig. 1. Illustrated convolutional neural network. Example of vehicle image classification. Source: Towards Data Science.

The construction of the network will be done using the Keras library, which belongs to Tensorflow. This library facilitates the user's process of training deep learning models, as it contains a variety of previously validated "Deep learning frameworks" [12]. One of the advantages of this library is its ability to build robust models from relatively small datasets (less than 1000 samples per class).

Some useful features of Keras are the following:

- **Fit_generator**. It performs neural network training. It depends on the next parameters: epoch, steps per epoch, batches and batch size. Although they are modifiable, the most relevant are not those mentioned, but the learning rate and the error and validation training, which define the quality of the model.
- **ImageDataGenerator**. This module generates more images using the original input images. To achieve this, it performs zooming, re-cutting, brightness alteration and other modifications in order to expand our original dataset and provide robustness to the model. All image transformation paramters are controllable, allowing to set a ratio in which the module will randomly modify the image. For example, you can configure the rotation range within which the image will be randomly rotated (see Fig. 2).

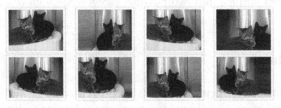

Fig. 2. This is what our data augmentation strategy looks like. Source: The Keras Blog.

Finally, you must set the number of classes in which you want to classify the image in keras. Each class must have three sets of images: training, validation and test. It is important that these 3 sets are mutually exclusive. In the training set are the data that will train the model. The validation set is used to prevent overfitting. The test set is used only to verify the validity of the model.

In the industrial field, the image classification is intended to be incorporated into a complete machine vision system, which contains the following components:

a) Object
b) Image sensor (camera)
c) Lighting
d) Image processing module
e) Decision module (software)

The list of components of such a system may vary depending on the source consulted. This is an adaptation without omission of other proposed systems [13].

Figure 3 successfully illustrates an example of a machine vision system.

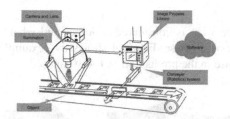

Fig. 3. Diagram of a machine vision system. Source: Innomiles International.

Image processing consists of 3 stages: smoothed, edge detection, enhancement.

Smoothed. At this stage the "Median Blur" filter from the OpenCV library is used. This filter is classified as a smoothed filter and its purpose is to reduce the noise in the images, which is useful to facilitate the conservation and edge detection [14]. The filter acts on the entire image and replaces the value of each pixel with the average value of the surrounding pixels within a defined radius. The only parameter that can be manipulated is the radius of the filter.

Edge Detection. The combination of the Sobel and Laplace operators, both of which are designed for edge detection, has been used before and has proven to be efficient and compatible with each other [15], allowing sharp changes in the original image to be successfully highlighted. Using a combination of two different edge detection filters is an unpopular technique, although very detailed results can be achieved.

One of the recognized edge detection operators is the so-called "Sobel Filter", which produces an image that emphasizes the edges of the original. The use of this filter has become widespread in image processing and machine vision [16].

The Laplace Operator is the second operator in the combination.

Enhancement. The last stage of digital image processing is an image enhancement using the Pillow library, available in Python. The "Contour" filter is used, which gives us a negative of the input image and improves the contours of the input image.

This image processing is sufficient to be used in the training of the neural network, since the result is a binary image that highlights only the relevant contours (edges of the piece and defects within it).

3 Dataset

In order to obtain a sample of significant size for later analysis, a footwear production workshop located in the city of León, Guanajuato, was contacted.

The workshop was asked for a wide variety of leather samples, composed of elements in good condition and elements with defects.

The sample consists of 92 different sheets of leather, among which the defects are predominant, which will be described below.

3.1 Defects

It is important to define what is considered a defect and what is not, in addition to the possible repercussions of these. Figure 4 shows two examples of leather in good condition, suitable for use in the production of footwear.

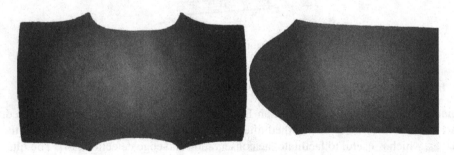

Fig. 4. Samples of leather without defects.

This leather has the characteristic of not containing wrinkles, folds, scars or holes on its surface. The absence of these defects allows its proper handling in the production process of footwear.

In Fig. 5, we find examples of the different defects present in the sample. In this case, no more types of defects were present, which presents an opportunity to expand the sample in order to obtain a more robust model.

It is important to remember that the presence of these defects may or may not be harmful depending on the type of product being manufactured. For the footwear industry in particular, the absence of these defects over a wide area is of great importance, since the leather will be subjected to processes of tension that the material will probably not

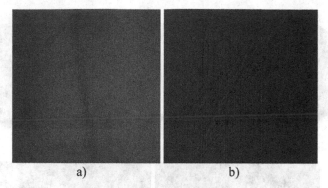

Fig. 5. Common defects in leather: a) Scars b) Creases.

be able to withstand if any of the defects are present. It may happen that the matte leather will resist the whole procedure, although this is even worse, since the final product will have a poor quality and a life span notably less than the expected.

3.2 Obtaining Samples

As mentioned, the leather samples were provided by a shoe workshop located in the city of Leon, Guanajuato. The digitalization process consisted in taking pictures using a Samsung S5KGM1 sensor with 48-megapixel resolution.

The capture of photographs was done in a clean space, so that the sensor captured only the leather sheet. An LED lamp (or any other direct light source) is needed to continuously illuminate the leather samples, so that the picture is clear and easy to process.

4 Procedure

Once the dataset is built, the next step is the digital processing of images.

For this, the OpenCV and scikit-learn libraries, both available in Python, were used. In comparison to other researches, a combination of different filters was used, so that they could highlight the information related to the defects and at the same time reduce the information that is not useful for the analysis of the images.

With the processed images the next step is to build a convolutional neural network.

For this purpose, the Keras library, which belongs to Tensorflow.

4.1 Image Processing

Figure 6 shows an image processing results, allowing to buy between the original and the processed image, as well as the sample of leather with defects and without defects.

The Median Blur filter, available in the OpenCV library, was used. The only modifiable parameter is the radius of pixels used for averaging. The larger this radius is, the

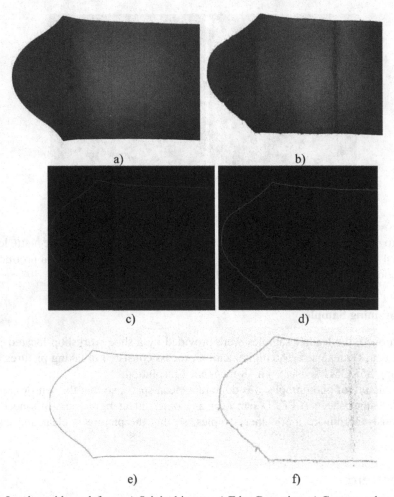

Fig. 6. Leather without defects: a) Original image, c) Edge Detection, e) Contour enhancement. Leather with defects: b) Original image, d) Edge Detection, f) Contour enhancement.

less sharp the image is. This filter allows us to get rid of noise and irrelevant information present in the image.

Later, we used the combination of operators "Sobel Filter" and "Laplace Operator", belonging to the Scikit-learn and OpenCV libraries, respectively. The benefits of this combination were described previously and the result can be seen in Fig. 6(c and d).

Finally, we applied the "Contour" filter from the Pillow library, which gives us a negative of the image and an enhancement in the contours, as shown in Fig. 6(e and f).

4.2 Neural Network Training

To develop the image classification system, a convolutional neural network was trained using TensorFlow's "Keras" library, whose operation and validity were developed in the "Fundamentals" section.

The network was configured so that the training consists of 20 epochs, with a learning rate of 0.0004 and a minimum accuracy of 75%. Raising any of these parameters (reducing in the case of the learning rate) offers a better-quality training, although this requires a computer with better performance than that available (especially on the GPU) and long waiting times, so it was decided to keep this.

5 Results

The Keras library provides us with information on the result of the training, which was 80% accurate. To measure the validity and check the reliability of the model built, the data set called test set is used, which consists of 20 images, 10 of them of leather in good condition and 10 of leather with defects, in order to check if the model is able to classify them correctly. It is important to clarify that the test images cannot be the same ones used to train the network. The results of this test are focused on Table 1.

Table 1. Results of model predictions.

Image description	Test samples	Correct predictions
Flawless leather	10	7
Flawed leather	10	10
Total	20	17

The model works well in detecting errors, as it successfully sorts out images showing defective leather parts. However, only 7 out of 10 images made an accurate prediction. This means that the system would potentially reject 30% of the samples that are in good condition. However, it would be able to identify an error 100% of the time. Overall, the system seems to make predictions with an 85% effectiveness.

6 Future Work

At least 3 next steps are easily identifiable after the completion of this paper.

Improvement. The first step is to improve the model. To do this, it is strictly necessary to extend the data set used, to perform a strict sampling of at least 2000 samples and with a greater variety of defects. In addition, the image processing can also be optimized compared to that used in other projects of a similar nature.

Artificial Vision System. The second step consists of adding the code to a complete artificial vision system. Since it is written in Python and can be quickly co-written in the cloud, a Raspberry Pi would be ideal to reduce implementation costs. It would also require the placement of a conveyor belt, direct lighting and RGB LED lights or speaker for an alarm to notify that an error was detected.

Implementation. The last step is the implementation of the system in a shoe production workshop, provided that the model has proved useful. A demonstration would be made to the managers to allow them to verify that the system works with reduced margins of error, so that they feel confident to automate the inspection process.

7 Conclusion

Image processing and neural network training using Keras and Tensorlow with a small data set is a potentially useful tool in the area of quality control and machine vision.

Although the trained model presents weaknesses in the identification of parts without defects, the percentage is high enough to consider it a useful option, highlighting that it is obviously subject to improvement and making it clear that as further work the data set to be processed must be greatly expanded.

The processing of the images is also subject to improvement, different combinations of filters could offer better results.

The image processing, the convolutional neural network training and the prediction system were executed in the cloud using the Google Colab platform, which supports Python. Also, Python is the most widely used language in the Raspberry Pi ordinances, frequently used in the Internet of Things. These facts give a better perspective to systems like this, since the inclusion in a production line using Raspberry Pi and wireless network modules, as well as the ability to work in the cloud, imply a large area of implementation opportunity at low cost, provided that it is done with the necessary knowledge.

References

1. Pacheco Vega, R.: Historia de dos ciudades: un análisis comparativo de los distritos industriales del cuero y calzado en León y Guadalajara. In: Meeting of the Latin American Studies Association (2004)
2. INEGI: Estadísticas a propósito de la Industria del calzado, México (2014)
3. Footwear - worldwidel Statista Market Forecast. https://www.statista.com/out-look/110 00000/100/footwear/worldwide
4. Perng, D., Liu, H., Chang, C.: Automated SMD LED inspection using machine vision. Int. J. Adv. Manuf. Technol. **57**, 1065–1077 (2011)
5. Aguilar-Torres, M., Argüelles-Cruz, A., Yánez-Márquez, C.: A real time artificial vision implementation for quality inspection of industrial products. In: 2008 Electronics, Robotics and Automotive Mechanics Conference, pp. 277–282 (2008)
6. Wu, M., Phoha, V.V., Moon, Y.B., Belman, A.K.: Detecting malicious defects in 3D Printing Process Using Machine Learning And Image Classification. In: ASME 2016 International Mechanical Engineering Congress and Exposition (2016)

7. Armesto, L., Tornero, J., Herraez, A., Asensio, J.: Inspection system based on artificial vision for paint defects detection on cars bodies. In: 2011 IEEE International Conference on Robotics and Automation, pp. 1–4. IEEE (2011)
8. Gnanavel, S., Manohar, S., Sridhar, K., Sokkanarayanan, S., Sathiyanarayanan, M.: Quality detection of fresh fruits and vegetables to improve horticulture and agro-industries. In: 2019 International Conference on contemporary Computing and Informatics (IC3I), pp. 268–272 (2019)
9. Bong, H., Truong, Q., Nguyen, H., Nguyen, M.: Vision-based inspection system for leather surface defect detection and classification. In: 2018 5th NAFOSTED Conference on Information and Computer Science (NICS), pp. 300–304 (2018)
10. Liong, S.T., et al.: Efficient neural network approaches for leather defect classification. arXiv preprint. (2019)
11. Simard, P., Steinkraus, D., Platt, J.: Best practices for convolutional neural networks applied to visual document analysis. In: Seventh International Conference on Document Analysis and Recognition, vol. 3 (2003)
12. Nandy, A., Biswas, M.: Reinforcement learning with keras, tensorflow, and chainerrl. In: Reinforcement Learning, pp. 129–153 (2017)
13. Liu, B., Wu, S., Zou, S.: Automatic detection technology of surface defects on plastic products based on machine vision. In: 2010 International Conference on Mechanic Automation and Control Engineering, pp. 2213–2216 (2010)
14. Perreault, S., Hébert, P.: Median filtering in constant time. IEEE Trans. Image Process. 16(9), 2389–2394 (2007)
15. Gupta, S., Porwal, R.: Combining laplacian and sobel gradient for greater sharpening. ICTACT J. Image Video Process. 06, 1239–1243 (2016)
16. Jin-Yu, Z., Yan, C., Xian-Xiang, H.: Edge detection of images based on improved Sobel operator and genetic algorithms. In: 2009 International Conference on Image Analysis and Signal Processing, pp. 31–35 (2009)
17. Simard, P., Steinkraus, D., Platt, J.: Best practices for convolutional neural networks applied to visual document analysis. In: Seventh International Conference on Document Analysis and Recognition, 2003, vol. 3 (2003)

Suppliers Analysis and Selection to Improve Supply Chain Performance

Inaivis L. Ibañez-Delgado(✉), Tomás E. Salais-Fierro, and Jania A. Saucedo-Martinez

Universidad Autónoma de Nuevo León, Pedro de Alba S/N, Niños Héroes, Ciudad Universitaria, San Nicolás de los Garza, Nuevo León, Mexico
inaidelgado93@gmail.com, tomas.salaisfr@uanl.edu.mx, jania.saucedo@gmail.com

Abstract. Having good suppliers not only means having quality supplies, it also means having low costs. Suppliers play a fundamental role in the production process from the acquisition of raw materials and even in the design and innovation of products. After an analysis of the literature related to the objective of the research, this article proposes a methodology for the analysis and selection of suppliers in order to improve the performance of the supply chain and also to be able to face the diversity and complexity of the situations that may arise in the purchasing process. The article provides professionals with flexibility and effectiveness in the selection of suppliers and their selection process, and with a better understanding of their future purchasing strategies. The fundamental findings of this research focus specifically on the determination and analysis of the main methods quantitative used in the selection of the supplier. The proposed methodology is applied in a company in the automotive sector and there is a good expectation of the methodology since in the preliminary investigations satisfactory results have been obtained.

Keywords: Suppliers · Supply chain · Selection process · Quantitative methods

1 Introduction

Nowadays, internationally successful companies are supplying the world's best competitive advantages [1], making it vitally important for them to develop competitive strategies based on value aggregation and simultaneous cost reduction [2]. As well as integrated management of supply-manufacturing-distribution tertiary and effective integration into international marketing networks [3]. For that reason, suppliers and customers must be partners in supply chains and not be faced with isolated authorities. Having good suppliers can not only mean having quality inputs and, therefore, being able to offer quality products, but also these give companies the possibility of having low costs, or the security of always having the same products whenever they are required [4]. In the case of the automotive sector, suppliers play a fundamental role in the process from the acquisition of raw materials to even the design and innovation of products.

© ICST Institute for Computer Sciences, Social Informatics and Telecommunications Engineering 2021
Published by Springer Nature Switzerland AG 2021. All Rights Reserved
J. A. Marmolejo-Saucedo et al. (Eds.): COMPSE 2020, LNICST 359, pp. 62–85, 2021.
https://doi.org/10.1007/978-3-030-69839-3_5

According to the analyzed literature, within the common problems, as a result of the poor selection of suppliers in the automotive sector, approximately 43% are associated with supply problems, therefore, our study will focus on this problem. The deficiency in supply in a factor that negatively affects the production process by increasing its variability and increasing the risks of obtaining a product without the spices requested by the customer [5]. Inadequate supplier selection could also have a negative impact by bringing with it increased costs, late deliveries of products, incomplete deliveries and elongation of cycles [6]. The objective of this article is to propose a methodology for the analysis and selection of suppliers within the automotive sector to improve the performance of the supply chain. In order to comply with our objective, it is essential to investigate about the processes for the selection of suppliers, which methodology has been used in the literature, as well as what criteria have been managed and which tools have been developed.

Supplier selection should have as its main criterion the ability of the supplier to improve and work under collaborative policies, without neglecting the characteristics traditionally valued such as price, quality, delivery time and payment plans [7]. Supplier selection is a multi-criteria problem, which includes quantitative and qualitative factors [8], so to select the best supplier it is necessary to make compensation between several factors. It is not easy to make the decision about which is the best supplier and therefore methodologies have been developed to help in this process.

For the supplier selection process, [9] proposes that firstly, the problems and objectives pursued by the company must be identified. Then, to determine the selection criteria according to the entity's own needs and later to select and apply a selection method.

There are multiple criteria to consider for the selection of the right suppliers for the logistics process of companies. They range from presenting attractive prices of the products, raw materials, or services they provide, delivery at the necessary time and to providing a quick response to some inconvenience. In a complex decision environment such as that surrounding supply chain management, cost- and price decisions proposed by the supplier are somewhat dangerous if they are not based on a comprehensive analysis of the economic context, existing restrictions and dominant business practices such as thorough market research [10]. For this reason, the complexity of a supply process should consider a set of variables related to transport, market fluctuations, costs, quality requirements, negotiation processes and inspection procedures.

Once the criteria are identified, the next step is to choose the suppliers by applying a certain method. The selection method must be consistent with the analysis of the context, the realities of the supply chain the selected criteria. Depending on the method selected, the efficiency of the purchase decision can be increased by enabling faster and more automated processing of data, eliminating redundant criteria and alternatives in decision-making processes, and facilitating more effective communication [11]. In the literature we can find referenced several methods that have been used for the selection of suppliers. These can be classified or grouped into Mathematical Methods, Statistical Methods, Artificial Intelligence Methods, and Integrated Methods which is the combination of 2 or more methods from the above classifications [12].

This article is organized as follows. The next section will discuss the background of the investigation where it will be presented, among other things, what methodologies they have used for the selection of suppliers, the main selection criteria, as well as the tools used. Subsequently as a conclusion we will analyze the methodology that we propose in this article.

2 Background

Within this field of supplier management, a significant number of contributions are in the specialized literature that are oriented to the development of three fundamental topics: (1) supplier management as part of supply chain management, (2) suppliers selection as a strategic decision and (3) techniques and methods to support the decision to select suppliers [7].

The management of an efficient supplier system as a link in the supply chain is considered one of the most impact and complex logistical tools in sourcing operations in companies. Supplier management is a key element in the modern administration of organizations, especially when the quality of what enters the process is considered to affect the quality of the outputs, which is a potential when it comes to improving the purchasing system associated with efficient supply chains [11]. For this reason, it is essential that companies have a process of selection of suppliers that analyze different aspects that result in the selection of the best partner.

2.1 Methodologies for Supplier Selection Processes

For decades, researchers and professionals from various branches have paid close attention to the selection of suppliers and the methods to be able to select them properly. Supplier selection is a multi-crime problem, which includes quantitative and qualitative factors. To select the best supplier, it is necessary to make a compensation between these tangible and intangible factors between which there may be conflict [11]. It is not easy to make the decision about which is the best supplier and therefore methodologies have been developed to help in this process.

In the case of Vírseda, 2011 [9], it proposes a supplier selection process comprising 4 fundamental steps: Assessing needs and defining objectives; Gather a group of suppliers; Interview with suppliers; Select and apply a method.

In the first step in assessing the company's needs and the corresponding requirements for contacting the appropriate suppliers, it proposes that a list should be created with the selection criterias that are taken to evaluate suppliers. The second step of bringing together a group of suppliers is to be done through a "request for information" (RFI) to learn more about these companies, as well as through previous market research. Once all the proposals are received from the suppliers, the company makes a technical and commercial evaluation. Each company uses a different way of evaluating and selecting suppliers through different methods. Finally, a supplier is selected, and the terms of delivery and service are negotiated.

On the other hand, [13] emphasizes that the vendor selection process can include several stages such as the following:

1. Recognize the need for supplier selection, i.e. determine what factors have been presented in companies that have led to problems in the entity.

2. Identifying key requirements of those depends on business objectives.
3. Determine sources of supply or supplier selection criteria.
4. Limit suppliers in selection group or what is the same, determine a portfolio of suppliers.
5. Determine the method of evaluation and selection of the supplier.
6. Select vendor and make an agreement.

The methodology proposed by [14] is also robust, because it defines different steps for the supplier selection process that take into account the diversity and complexity of the situations that may arise in the purchasing process and the importance of taking it in bill.

The four stages defined by Boer [14] are as follows:

a) Defining the problem
b) Determination of the attributes to be evaluated
c) Evaluation of suppliers using a technique and
d) Final selection of the supplier.

As for the definition of the problem, the author argues that it is necessary to understand the problem through certain questions such as: What is the life cycle of the product or component? Why is there a need to select a new provider? What have been the problems you have had with previous suppliers? To determine the attributes to be evaluated the author proposes that they can be classified into quantitative attributes (which can be measured by a previously established scale), or qualitative attributes (cannot be expressed by a unit or measurement scale so evaluation and experience of people who know the problem is required). These attributes or criteria must be selected according to the needs of the company. Once the criteria are defined, the next step is to choose suppliers by applying a certain method that must be consistent with the analysis of the context, the realities of the supply chain and the selected criteria.

2.2 Supplier Selection Criteria

As discussed in the previous section and in the examples above, one of the main aspects of the vendor selection process is the selection criteria.

The selection of suppliers constitutes a strategic decision with a high impact on the performance of the organization, for this reason it is considered necessary to select the right supplier, in favor of strategic development and according to the specific needs of the company [15]. Resources are directed only to working with those suppliers with whom we can obtain significant and valuable value [4].

There are multiple criteria to be able to select the right suppliers for the logistics process of companies. They range from presenting attractive prices of the products, raw materials, or services they provide, to providing a quick response to some inconvenience. In a complex decision-making environment, decisions based only on the price proposed by the supplier and costs are somewhat dangerous if they are not based on a comprehensive analysis of the economic context, existing restrictions and dominant business practices [7]. An important point to note is that some criteria are often in conflict with each other, as the increase of one characteristic may mean the decrease of another [11].

Each of these aspects must be selected according to the needs of the business, i.e. they are inherent to each product supplied and are of great importance within the selection model. In literature and in practice, the most used criterias for supplier selection are quality, sales price, and delivery times, however, there are many other criteria within these criteria we cite the following:

- Certified quality management system: The supplier must demonstrate its ability to establish, document and implement an effective quality management system.
- Administrative capacity: The main thing is that suppliers have administrative maturity that allows them to establish a cooperative and society relationship based on maintaining optimal levels of quality, costs and services.
- Business performance: The company requires a supplier that is profitable for it, in terms of discounts and payment terms. This aspect, typical of each supplier, demonstrates its commercial stability and provides a confidence support in economic terms.
- Financial stability: Suppliers have a stable and sound financial position, which is a good indicator when making long-term negotiations.
- Treatment of complaints and complaints: The supplier must develop effective strategies to resolve complaints and concerns, investigate their causes and therefore improve the service provided to the company on an ongoing basis.
- Geographical positioning, distribution centers and technical support: The entity must have efficient suppliers, considering that geographical positioning can influence delivery times, cost in freight-insurance and legal documentation.
- Processing of information in online order handling: Suppliers must have a reliable information handling system to observe the compliance status of purchase orders, shipments and inventory system. You need to select suppliers that are related to the research and development of your products and services.
- Installed production capacity: Knowing capacity is essential for business management as it allows to analyze the degree of use of each of the resources in the organization and thus can optimize them.
- Technical Product Specifications: The supplier must ensure that the product you provide meets all specifications included in the purchase order. Material certifications containing the results measured during production are required.
- Sales price: Suppliers are required to have stable behavior in relation to the fluctuation in the price of the products offered and in addition that the prices provided by the supplier are competitive according to the market.
- Logistics performance: Each supplier must ensure that logistics development activities are planned and carried out during the stages of the product lifecycle, thus ensuring the satisfaction of the specifications requested by the company in all aspects [7, 11].

On the other hand, supplier selection should have as its main criterion the ability of the supplier to improve and work under collaboration policies, without regard to the characteristics assessed above, among others. Logically, not all attributes are equally important to all companies. As mentioned above, each company is a special case that presents its own needs and that can face different problems (Molamohamadi et al. [16]).

3   Quantitative Methods Used for Supplier Selection

Another fundamental aspect of the supplier selection process is to choose them by applying a method. This, once the criteria are identified. The selection method must be consistent with the analysis of the context, the realities of the supply chain and the selected criteria.

It is recurring then to know some of the tools or methods that have been used in this regard. The techniques used for vendor selection in general can be classified or grouped into Mathematical Methods, Statistical Methods, Artificial Intelligence Methods, and Integrated Methods which is the combination of two or more methods from the above classifications. Will be analyzed some of these methods below.

3.1   Mathematical Methods

For a long time, the methods that have been used most for the selection of suppliers are mathematical methods, since the main objective of numerical analysis is to find "approximate" solutions to complex problems using only arithmetic operations. In this section we introduce some of these techniques.

Analytic Hierarchy Process (AHP)
Within Mathematical Methods, the Analytical Hierarchy Process or AHP is one of the most widely discussed methods in both supplier selection and general. It was introduced by [17],and is a measurement theory that provides the ability to incorporate both qualitative and quantitative factors into the decision-making process. It therefore facilitates decision-making by organizing criteria or judgments into a hierarchical multi-level structure that exhibits the forces influencing a decision [18]. [19] define AHP as a decision-making method for prioritizing alternatives when multiple criteria should be used. In addition, we can say that the AHP generates numerical priorities based on subjective criteria and organizes them into paired comparison matrices. His greatest strength lies in his ability to hierarchically structure a complex, multi-goal problem and then investigate each level of hierarchy separately [7]. From the analyzed literature, it can be said that this is the most used quantitative tool for the suppliers' selection.

Linear Programming (LP)
Linear programming has also been used in this field. It is a widely used methodology based on mathematical models and sometimes complex systems of equations. It was created to give a practical and resource optimization sense in the quest to obtain a better and more concrete solution, as is the case in the allocation and distribution of resources when these are limited [20]. We can also say that Linear Programming is a technique that is used to optimize a function subject to constraints, this with the aim of identifying possible results or combinations for the best decision [21]. In other words, Linear Programming is an optimization method in the sense of reaching a more

appropriate result. It then aims to solve problems and determine the best combination of activities to optimize resources and use only what is necessary, this technique is designed to support managers in planning and decision-making [22].

Goal Programming (GP)

Goal Programming is in a linear programming extension to deal with problems with multiple, usually conflicting targets. It allows decision makers to set their suction levels for each target [23]. It is also the most widely used approach in the field of decision-making with multiple criteria that allows the decision-maker to incorporate numerous variations of constraints and objectives and aims to minimize the deviation between the achievement of the objectives and their aspiration. It can be said that GP has been, the most widely used multi-goal technique in management science due to its inherent flexibility in managing decision-making problems with various objectives to be addressed [24].

Data Envelopment Analysis (DEA)

Data Envelopment Analysis is another mathematical method used for supplier selection, it is a mathematical linear programming technique that calculates the relative efficiency of multiple decision-making units, based on multiple inputs and multiple outputs, without needing to know any functional relationship between them. DEA is based on the concept of efficiency of a decision alternative. Alternatives are evaluated in terms of cost-benefit ratio [11]. According to De Boer [14], efficiency is measured from the value ranging from the average sum of profits to the values of the cost criteria. This method allows suppliers to be classified into two initial categories: efficient suppliers or inefficient vendors. This tool can be applied in multipurpose troubleshooting.

Simulation

Simulation is another mathematical method used for supplier selection, which to a lesser extent. Simulation is a tool whereby both new and existing processes can be projected, evaluated and contemplated without risk, associated with experiences carried out in a real system. In other words, it allows organizations to study their processes from a systematic perspective by seeking a better understanding of the cause and effect between them in addition to allowing a better prediction of certain situations [25]. Simulation models can be classified into Static, Dynamic, Deterministic, Stochastic, Discrete, Continuous, Physical, Analog, or Symbolic [14, 26]. For supply chain optimization professionals, a major difficulty is the uncertainty and dynamics that occur along supply chain, therefore simulation, due to its ability to handle variability, is a very popular tool for these systems. Discrete event simulation is one of the most widely used and accepted tools in supply chain analysis [27].

Preference Ranking Organization Method for Enrichment Evaluation (PROMETHEE)

PROMETHEE is a method for evaluating alternatives to decision-making with multiple criteria. It is characterized by many types of preference functions that are used to assign differences between alternatives in trials [28]. We can also say that PROMETHEE is a classification method that is considered simple in conception and calculation compared to many other multicriteria decisions methods. It is well adapted to decision problems where a finite set of alternatives must be exceeded subject to multiple criteria [29] and is based on peer comparisons of alternatives with respect to each criterion. It is also a method that can be applied to real-life planning problems such as business, government institutions, transportation, health care and education [28]. In short, PROMETHEE helps decision makers find the alternative that best suits their goal and understanding of the problem. It provides an integral and rational framework for structuring a decision problem, identifying and quantifying its conflicts and associations, working groups, and highlighting the main alternatives with structured reasoning [30].

3.2 Statistical Methods

Cluster Analysis
In this respect we should point out Cluster Analysis, which is a very important technology. Its primary goal is to divide a large amount of unprocessed data into multiple groups according to evaluation rules so managers can use split groups for decision making. The purpose is to differentiate the grouped data by calculating similarities between data or following other evaluation rules so that differentiated data can form multiple groups that are characterized by high similarity of data in the same group. Supplier cluster analysis is an important procedure in building a supply chain system as selecting the right supplier group could strengthen operational capacity and reduce business risks [31].

3.3 Artificial Intelligence Methods

Artificial Intelligence (AI) is one of the branches of computer science that has aroused the most interest today, due to its huge field of application. The search for mechanisms that help us understand intelligence and make models and simulations of them, is something that has motivated many scientists to choose this area of research.

Artificial Neural Networks
Among the Artificial Intelligence methods used in the literature for the suppliers' selection is Artificial Neural Network. These are but an artificial and simplified model of the human brain, which is the best example that we have for a system that is able to acquire knowledge through experience, that is to reproduce certain characteristics typical of humans, such as the ability to memorize and associate facts. A neural network is a new system for the treatment of information, whose basic processing unit is inspired by the fundamental cell of the human nervous system: the neuron [32]. Therefore, Neural Networks consist of processing units that exchange data or information, are used to recognize patterns, including images, manuscripts, and time sequences (e.g. financial trends). They can learn and improve their functioning [33].

Analytic Network Process (ANP)
Another mathematical method that has been used in the literature for supplier selection is the Analytic Network Process, which is a generalization of the AHP and can be used to treat more sophisticated decision problems than AHP [11]. The ANP provides a general

framework for handling decisions without assuming about the independence of the top-level elements of the lower-level elements and on the independence of elements within a level. Therefore, ANP is represented by a network without the need to specify levels as in a hierarchy [19]. The elements of the network influence each other, which the decider values by paired comparisons whose intensity is measured on Saaty's 1–9 scale. [11]. In other words, by using the ANP, we can model dependencies and feedback between decision-making elements, and calculate more accurate criteria weights and local and global alternative priorities [17].

Fuzzy Set Theory (FST)
In the literature we can also find a method called Fuzzy Set Theory (FST), which allows to represent common knowledge, which is mostly of the qualitative linguistic type and not necessarily quantitative, in a mathematical language [11]. This method should be used to process inaccurate data and inaccurate information obtained from complex situations that cannot reasonably be described in conventional quantitative expressions [34]. Therefore, FST allows a generalization of the concept of classic set for modeling complex and poorly defined systems. The main concepts associated with FST, as applied to membership functions, linguistic variable, natural language computing; arithmetic operations of fuzzy sets and fuzzy weighted average, among others [35].

Case Based Reasoning (CBR)
Another method is Case Based Reasoning. This is an administrative software system by a database that collects relevant information from decision-making processes and evaluation of previously occurred situations or cases. In this way the decision maker can rely on useful information and experiences of known situations. The CBR allows for successful procurement management, as it has the advantage that by taking into account the progress made in previous processes, it does not give room for the same mistakes to be made again, especially because it reuses relevant information in evaluations that suppliers have made previously [11]. In other words, a CBR system is a software-based database that provides useful information and experiences from previous decision-maker situations like a decision maker [14].

Expert System (ES)
Expert System is one of the successful fields of application in Artificial Intelligence. It is a knowledge-based system that uses an inference procedure to solve problems that would otherwise require human competence or experience. The power of expert systems comes primarily from specific knowledge about a narrow domain stored in the knowledge base. Therefore, expert systems use human knowledge to simulate expert performance, and present a human facade to users. Expert systems can advise, instruct and assist humans in decision-making, justify a conclusion and suggest alternatives to a problem [36].

As mentioned above, these are some of the methods that have been used for vendor selection. The integration of several methods discussed above has also been used for this. A summary of these is referenced in the Table 1.

On the other hand, it is important to point out some problems that have arisen within organizations due to the inadequate supplier's selection. Such as the financial problems, operation of the logistics system, deficiency in the supply of raw materials and supplies

Table 1. Methods used for supplier selection

Methods		Authors
Mathematical	Analytic Hierarchy Process (AHP)	Yadav & Sharma (2014)
	Linear Programming (LP)	Talluri et al. (2005)
	Goal Programming (GP)	Azmi, & Tamiz (2014)
	Data Envelopment Analysis (DEA)	Garfamy (2006)
	PROMETEE	Abdullah et al. (2018)
	Simulation	Salmasnia et al. (2018)
Statistical	Cluster Analysis	Che & Wang (2009)
Artificial intelligence	Artificial neural networks (ANN)	Fernández et al. (2009)
	Case Based Reasoning (CBR)	Zhao & Yu (2011)
	Expert System (ES)	Chen et al. (2006)
	Fuzzy set Theory (FST)	Florez-Lopez (2007)
	Analytic Network Process (ANP)	Sarkis et al. (2002)
Integrated	AHP, DEA	Ramanathan (2007)
	AHP, GP	Kull et al. (2008)
	FUZZY, AHP	Kumar & Garg (2016)
	Simulation, DEA	Azadeh & Zarrin (2014)
	Artificial neural networks, AHP, DEA	Ha et al. (2008)

for production, delivery of defective and incomplete products or inadequate services and loss of customers by not following up on claims, among others that may arise.

Within the analyzed literature that deals with the topic of provider analysis and selection, the most used method is AHP, however, other methods such as ANP, Neural Networks and integrated methods have also been recently used by authors and researchers. Although in the coming years it is to be expected the use of many more tools for the development of investigations

In order to argue the above, in the Table 2 has been drawn up with some of the researchers who have addressed the topic of supplier selection, the problems that have been developed, the methods used for the solution of the same, as well as the benefits they provided.

Table 2. Relationship of some problems derived from the inadequate selection of suppliers in the automotive sector, some authors and the methods used.

Authors	Methods	Problems	Advantage
Galankashi, MR et al. (2016)	AHP, FUZZY	Finance	Flexibility for attribute selection and weighted judgment on the importance of criteria
Gómez, J. C. et al. (2008)	AHP	Deficiencies in the operation of the logistics system	Weight scoring method is used to select critical criteria and suppliers
Tafernaberri Franzão, E. (2018)	ANP	Late delivery of contracted products or services	The article has proposed a multi-perspective approach framework for provider selection
Yadav. V & Sharma. M (2015)	AHP	Product delivery defective and/or incomplete or inadequate services	The proposed model can handle many suppliers. Furthermore, it does not require any special programming or complex computational efforts
Perçin, S. (2006)	AHP, LP	Deficiencies in the supply of raw materials and inputs for production	To consider quantitative and qualitative factors in selecting the best suppliers and assigning optimal order quantities among them
Kar, A (2015)	AHP, FUZZY, ANN	Loss of customers by not following up on claims	To determine the optimal order of quantities to be allocated to multiple suppliers under consideration of additional restrictions. Models can be used to automate workflow, to maintain supplier records, and to standardize evaluation and order allocation processes

4   Discussion

Procurement management to be considered a true source of competitive advantage within the supply chain requires more efficient logistics processes. Its strategy should be aligned with the business strategy and with the overall objectives of competitiveness; therefore, procurement targets should be set based on a set of criteria, such as cost, quality, delivery time, service, among others. In many cases these criteria make the selection of supplier's complex, because most cases these criteria are of an eminent nature. Because the supplier's selection of in business management is so important, it is essential to find ways to try to eliminate subjectivity in the supplier selection process using specific tools. To achieve this, it is important to have a well-defined process or methodology that allows us to select the best supplier.

According to the different examples presented above, this article proposes a methodology for supplier selection with which we could appropriately select suppliers. The proposed methodology has four steps and its represented in the Fig. 1:

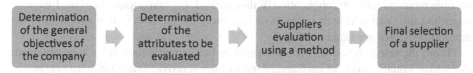

Fig. 1. Representation of the methodology

1. Determination of the general objectives of the company: At this stage you must carry out a trace of all those suppliers that can or present influence in the market that is located the company and for this purpose the managers of the purchasing department and the general management of the company must perform a series of questions and their respective analyses that will lead to greater clarity of the problem.
2. Determination of the attributes to be evaluated: These criteria or attributes must be chosen by the decision group or group of choice of the company. As well as through direct observations to the process consult the criteria that are used in the literature, which have already been analyzed in previous chapters. each company is a special case that presents its own needs and that can face different problems, the criteria must be selected according to these problems.
3. Evaluation of suppliers using a method: Once the selection criteria are defined, the next step is to select suppliers by applying a certain method. The selection method must be consistent with the analysis of the context, the realities of the supply chain and the selected criteria. As shown in the previous chapter, you can use an individual method or built-in methods, it all depends on what you want to get.
4. Final selection of a supplier: At this stage it is advisable that the decision group that has made the selection process, inform the senior management or senior managers of the company, in relation to the supplier that has been chosen, since it is they who must observe the attachment that this may have with the objectives and strategic plans that the company has.

5   Preliminary Results

The application of the proposed methodology will be carried out in the process of purchasing the Resin as one of the main raw materials used in the production of plastic products in a company that supplies these products to the automotive industry.

5.1   Determination of the General Objectives of the Company and Determination of the Attributes to Be Evaluated

The problem in this case study lies in the need to select the appropriate suppliers that can improve the performance of the procurement process of that company, cause the automotive sector is a very demanding one that requires there are not had any delays or product quality deficiencies because it can lead to very serious penalties.

To determine the critical indicators for the problem that concerns us and as part of the second step of the methodology, the Delphi Method was applied. This tool aims to obtain the most reliable consensus of opinions from a group of experts regarding a specific topic [37]. For the application of this method, the main opinions of the literature regarding the main attributes, criterias or indicators for the selection of suppliers in the automotive sector are taken.

From the research carried out, 45 criteria or fundamental indicators were obtained. For which a qualification of each one of the authors is provided according to exposed in their articles, using the scale with scores between 1 and 5. The results of the application of the method are shown in the tables where E1, E2, E3, E4, E5, E6, E7, E8, E9 and E10 represent the experts.

After analyzing the results of the application of the Delphi Method and using the Pareto Principle or also known as the 80/20 Rule, which establishes that the 80% of the consequences are derived from 20% of the causes; it can say that of the 45 criteria or indicators mentioned by the experts, the most important or critical criteria that represent approximately 20% of the total score are the following, in order of importance according to the percent they represent:

- Adequate quality of the supplies,
- certified Quality Management Systems,
- Adequate sale price,
- Minimum delivery times,
- Technological Capacity.

On the other hand, to check if there is agreement between the judgments of the experts regarding their selection in order to continue with the research, we will use a statistical tool called Kendall's Concordance Coefficient (W) (Table 3).

Kendall's coefficient of concordance (W) measures the degree of agreement between a group of elements (K) and a group of characteristics (n). It is commonly used in attribute agreement analysis. Kendall's coefficient values can range from 0 to 1. [38]. This statistician follows a Chi-square Distribution. For the development of this test two hypotheses are used:

Table 3. Result of the application of the Delphi Method

Delphi method											
Criterias	E1	E2	E3	E4	E5	E6	E7	E8	E9	E10	%
Quality of the supplies	5	5	5	5	5	5	5	5	5	5	0.0544
Certified quality management systems	5	4	5	4	4	5	4	4	4	4	0.0468
Sale price	4	4	5	3	5	5	4	5	1	5	0.0446
Minimum delivery times	4	4	5	4	4	1	1	5	5	5	0.0413
Technological capacity	1	5	5	3	5	5	4	4	5	1	0,0413
Total											0,2285

- Null hypothesis or H0: There is no agreement among the experts. $W = 0\ p > \alpha$
- Alternative hypothesis or H1: There is agreement among the experts. $W > 0\ p < \alpha$.

The Table 4 shows the value of the coefficient W with a significance level $\alpha = 0.05$ and $n = 5$ and degrees of freedom.

Table 4. Kendall's coefficient of concordance (W)

Kendal's coefficient			
W	Chi-square	DF	P
0,311940	12,4776	4	0,0141

Given that $W = 0.31194 > 0$ and $p = 0.0141 < 0.05$, H0 is rejected and H1 is accepted, therefore we can conclude that there is agreement between the experts. We will use the criterias: quality of the supplies, quality management systems, adequate sale price, minimum delivery times and technological capacity for the next steps of the proposed methodology.

5.2 Evaluation of Suppliers Using an Integrated Quantitative Method

After obtaining the criteria or indicators to evaluate, it proceeds to develop quantitative methods to select the appropriate supplier. For this case study, the managers and the Head of Purchasing have selected 5 suppliers, who have supplied the resin in the last year, a prior evaluation has been carried out on each supplier through a market investigation.

Analytic Hierarchy Process (AHP) Application

Firstly, for the supplier's evaluation, the Analytical Hierarchy Process or AHP will be developed. As previously mentioned, the AHP helps to make decisions in a more rational and understandable way. The AHP methodology for the development of this case is represented in Fig. 2.

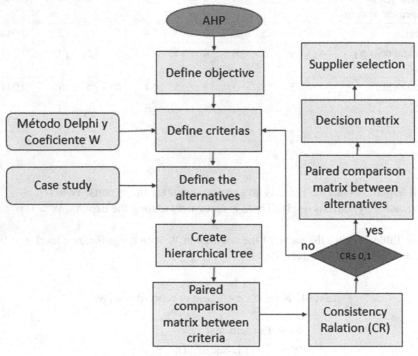

Fig. 2. AHP methodology

The inputs can be actual measurements, but also subjective opinions. Priorities or weightings and a consistency relationship will be calculated [21]. For the application of this method, the 5 criteria that were selected when applying the Delphi Method and the Kendall's Coefficient of Concordance and 5 alternatives or suppliers (S1, S2, S3, S4, S5).

As a first step in the application of the APH method, the paired comparison matrix should be made between the selected criteria A = [aij], where $1 \leq i, j \leq n$, for this, the experts or judges assign weights for each criterion with respect to the others using the Saaty Scale (1–9) (Table 5).

Table 5. Escala de Saaty

Intensity of importance aij	Definition	Explanation
1	Equal importance between i and j	The two criteria contribute the same to the objective
3	Little importance of element i over element j	Experience and judgment slightly favor one criterion over the other
5	Strong importance of element i over element j	Experience and judgment strongly favor one criterion over the other
7	Much stronger the importance of element i over element j	One criterion is favored very strongly over the other. In practice you can demonstrate your mastery
9	Absolute importance of element i over element j	The evidence favors one factor over the other to the highest degree

The paired comparison matrix between the selected criteria is shown in Table 6.

Table 6. Paired comparison matrix between criterias

Paired comparison matrix

	C1	C2	C3	C4	C5	Normalized matrix					Average vector
C1	1	5	5	1	5	0,38	0,66	0,41	0,29	0,24	0,40
C2	1/5	1	3	1	5	0,08	0,13	0,24	0,29	0,24	0,20
C3	1/5	1/3	1	1/3	3	0,08	0,04	0,08	0,10	0,14	0,09
C4	1	1	3	1	7	0,38	0,13	0,24	0,29	0,33	0,28
C5	1/5	1/5	1/3	1/7	1	0,08	0,03	0,03	0,04	0,05	0,04
SUM	2,60	7,53	12,33	3,48	21,00						

Subsequently, the alternatives are compared, that is, the 5 providers with respect to each of the 5 criteria. Therefore, comparison matrices of the alternatives are built according to each criterion and the proper or average vectors of each matrix are calculated (Table 7)

As our objective is to make a decision based on the 5 criteria and their importance, we proceed to multiply the matrices, one of them is composed of each of the weights of

Table 7. Average vectors of each supplier with respect to each criteria

	C1	C2	C3	C4	C5
S1	0,45	0,26	0,15	0,24	0,11
S2	0,15	0,22	0,11	0,17	0,22
S3	0,16	0,09	0,40	0,18	0,26
S4	0,07	0,09	0,10	0,19	0,12
S5	0,17	0,34	0,23	0,22	0,29

the alternatives based on each of the criteria and the other is the weighting of the criteria.

$$\begin{bmatrix} 0,45 \ 0,26 \ 0,15 \ 0,24 \ 0,11 \\ 0,15 \ 0,22 \ 0,11 \ 0,17 \ 0,22 \\ 0,16 \ 0,09 \ 0,40 \ 0,18 \ 0,26 \\ 0,07 \ 0,09 \ 0,10 \ 0,19 \ 0,12 \\ 0,17 \ 0,34 \ 0,23 \ 0,22 \ 0,29 \end{bmatrix} \times \begin{bmatrix} 0,40 \\ 0,20 \\ 0,09 \\ 0,28 \\ 0,04 \end{bmatrix} = \begin{bmatrix} 0,31 \\ 0,17 \\ 0,18 \\ 0,11 \\ 0,23 \end{bmatrix}$$

The final average vector indicates the weight of each alternative and therefore allows us to choose the best option. Based on the 5 criteria and their importance, the best alternative is Supplier 1 because it has the highest weight (0.31) followed by Supplier 5 (0.23), Supplier 3 (0.18), Supplier 2 (0.17) and finally the Supplier 4 (0.11).

Several analyzes can be carried out based on this result, from the need to make a systematic evaluation of the providers based on the criteria that were selected. Encourage and work together with the supplier 5 so that it can improve its performance in terms of a certified quality management system and that it complies to a greater extent with the quality specifications that are requested (since these are the highest criteria weight for decision makers in the company). To complement our decision, a model of artificial neural networks will be applied.

Artificial Neural Networks (ANN) Application
In this particular case study, another important element for which this neural network tool will be used is that our research is developed in the automotive industry and this industry is currently very demanding in terms of delivery, quality, logistics performance, provisioning, etc. As previously mentioned, artificial neural networks are used for prediction tasks and lead to an intelligent system that can successfully perform complex tasks. They can create patterns, recognize information, or solve complex problems.

The methodology to be followed for the development of neural networks in our case study is represented in the Fig. 3

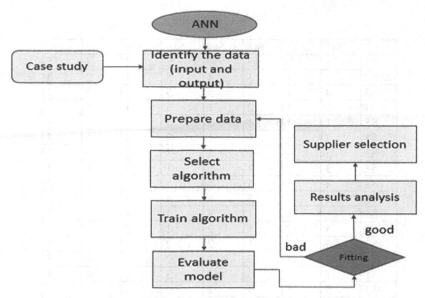

Fig. 3. ANN methodology

There are four aspects that characterize a neural network: its topology, type of association between the input and output information, the learning mechanism, and the form of representation of this information.

Particularly for our case study, which is a classification problem where there is input and output information, it will use the Feedforward Backpropagation network type, because a supervised learning mechanism is needed and this type of network is the most recommended for this kind of problems. Backpropagation networks have demonstrated their ability to work successfully in a wide range of applications including classification.

Particularly in our case study, the input data correspond to the evaluation of 5 suppliers for each of the 5 criteria in specifically 8 different stages that are the representative scenarios of our problem (40 suppliers) for a total of 200 input data, with a scale of 1–5 as follows, by the coordinating group of the company where the investigation was carried out:

1. Not at all satisfied with the supplier's performance
2. Not very satisfied with the supplier's performance
3. Neutral
4. Very satisfied with the supplier's performance
5. Totally satisfied with the supplier's performance (Table 8).

Table 8. Input data

	St1	St2	St3	St4	St5	St6	St7	St8
S1	5	5	3	4	5	2	3	5
S2	3	4	3	4	5	2	2	3
S3	4	1	2	3	5	2	4	2
S4	1	1	2	1	5	4	4	1
S5	1	1	1	1	3	5	4	4
S1	3	1	1	1	2	4	5	4
S2	3	3	4	5	1	3	5	4
S3	3	2	4	5	1	3	1	5
S4	4	4	4	5	5	5	1	2
S5	2	5	5	5	4	5	5	1
S1	1	1	1	4	4	4	5	3
S2	3	2	1	2	1	2	2	5
S3	3	4	1	2	2	1	3	5
S4	1	4	2	1	2	1	4	5
S5	2	5	3	2	3	1	4	4
S1	3	5	4	3	4	3	5	1
S2	2	5	4	3	5	3	5	2
S3	2	2	4	3	1	5	3	4
S4	2	1	5	1	1	5	4	5
S5	1	1	1	5	2	4	1	1
S1	3	2	2	5	4	2	2	5
S2	1	3	4	5	5	1	5	3
S3	2	4	5	5	3	1	5	2
S4	3	4	2	2	1	1	5	1
S5	5	5	2	2	1	5	5	5

The output data will correspond to the result of the application of the AHP for the 5 alternatives with respect to the 5 criteria, in the same stages (Table 9).

Table 9. Output data

AHP	S1	S2	S3	S4	S5	S6	S7	S8
S1	0,305	0,269	0,294	0,185	0,215	0,249	0,182	0,192
S2	0,168	0,217	0,183	0,189	0,175	0,144	0,182	0,187
S3	0,170	0,205	0,190	0,216	0,185	0,232	0,237	0,259
S4	0,120	0,121	0,163	0,237	0,255	0,197	0,233	0,190
S5	0,237	0,188	0,169	0,173	0,170	0,178	0,165	0,172

Another fundamental aspect are the network learning and training. Learning is the process by which a neural network modifies its weights in response to input information. The changes that occur during the learning stage are reduced to the destruction, modification and creation of connections between neurons.

For our training was used the Levenberg-Marquardt training function. This algorithm was developed in the early 1960s to solve online least squares problems. Least squares problems arise in the context of fitting a parameterized function to a set of measured data points by minimizing the sum of squares of the errors between the data points and the function n. The Levenberg-Marquardt algorithm combines two minimization methods: Gradient descent and the Gauss-Newton [39].

Two layers were also used to train our network, one of them hidden with 10 neurons in the hidden layer. As a performance function, the Mean Squared Error was used, and the Sigmoidal Function was used as the propagation function.

The software used for the training and simulation of the neural network was Matlab R2015a. After entering all the information mentioned above in the nntool tool of Matlab, we proceed to train the network, obtaining as a prototype of the neural network the one shown in Fig. 4.

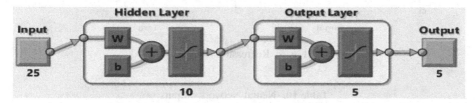

Fig. 4. Neural network's prototype

There are two fundamental aspects that the measurement gives us if the network is correctly trained or not. One of these is the Regression value (R), this value for both training, testing, validation and in general must be very close to 1, the closer to 1 that value is because the network will be better trained o in other terms good fitting. The resulting value of the regression is shown in Fig. 5 where it show that the value R = 0.99463, so that means that the network is good fitting.

Another aspect to consider is the accumulated error, in this case the algorithm must adjust the parameters of the network to minimize the mean square error. In this case the accumulated error was $1.25\ e^{-9}$ which represents a minimal error.

After the network is properly trained, it is simulated by entering the data that will be used for this purpose. In this case, 25 data were entered representing the evaluation of the five suppliers (analyzed for the AHP application) for each of the five criterias.

With all this information it proceeds to simulate the network. The output of the network corresponds to the weighting for each of the 5 suppliers (Table 10).

Through the network output, it shows that the supplier with the highest score is Supplier 1 (0.24305), so it is the selected provider. It is important to note that the output of the neural network corresponds to the result derived from the application of the AHP. For that reason, it means that the application of neural networks gives us more reliability to the result that it can obtain from the application of the AHP.

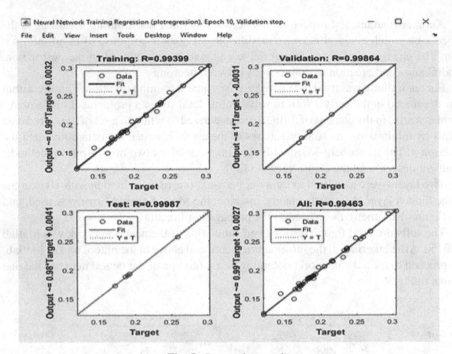

Fig. 5. Regression results

Table 10. Neural Network outputs

Suppliers	Weighting
1	0.24305
2	0.1673
3	0.171
4	0.12055
5	0.2311

5.3   Final Selection of a Supplier

Once the group of providers has been evaluated using the integrated AHP-ANN method, the next activity to perform is the final selection of the provider. At this stage it is convenient for the decision-making group that has carried out the selection process to inform the senior management or senior executives of the company, in relation to the supplier that has been chosen, since they are the ones who must observe the attachment that could have it with the objectives and strategic plans that the company has. It is possible that a decision made from an analytical point of view and based on a decision technique such as the previous ones, will be eliminated because it does not align with the strategic practices and plans of the company.

For this case the Supplier 1 complies in this aspect, which is why it was finally the selected supplier for providing the resin in the agreed period.

6 Conclusions

This study presents a procedure to analyze and select suppliers from an exhaustive search and the analysis of the academic literature related to methodologies or processes to properly select suppliers, selection criteria and even some of the quantitative methods that have been used. This article contributes to the supplier selection process and highlights the importance of supplier selection to improve the performance of the supply chain.

As part of the methodology, it can be concluded that the method choice phase is often the most visible phase of the process, however, the quality of this phase largely depends on the quality of the steps prior to that phase (Determination of the objectives of the company and determination of the attributes or criteria to evaluate). If buyers or decision makers strive to make sound decisions, they should also pay close attention to these first steps.

Also, our analysis showed that there are several criteria for selecting providers which can be objective or subjective. These criteria must be selected according to the environment and objectives of the company, in addition to the strategy that it has designed.

In addition, several of the methods that have been applied and that are useful for dealing with this problem were analyzed in this investigation. The allocation of methods must also be independent for each situation, since they all have different specific characteristics and purposes. The application of the correct method depends largely on the quality of the supplier selection process.

The proposed methodology was applied in a case study with the objective of selecting the appropriate supplier to supply resin for a company within the automotive sector. As important data, an integrated AHP-ANN method was used as a quantitative method to select the supplier, concluding that if a supplier can be obtained objectively, according to the needs of the company using said method.

References

1. Mcgraw-hill, A.E.: CAPÍTULO 3: Selección de proveedores (2008). http://webquery.ujmd. edu.sv/siab/bvirtual/Fulltext/ADPS0000636/C3.pdf
2. Acevedo Suarez, J.: Modelo de Gestión Integrada de la Cadena de Suministro, pp. 1–10 (2013)
3. Pyke, D.F., Johnson, M.E.: Sourcing strategy and supplier relationships: alliances vs. eProcurement forthcoming in the practice of supply chain management. In: Pract. Supply Chain Manag., pp. 77–89. Kluwer Publishers (2003)
4. Brien, J.O.: Supplier Relationship Management. Unlocking the Hidden Value in Your Supply Base. Kogan Page, London (2014)
5. Pavòn, S.C.: Sistema de aprovicionamiento para un programa de mantenimiento (2006)
6. Zubar, H.A., Parthiban, P.: Analysis of supplier selection methods through analytical approach. Int. J. Logist. Syst. Manag. 18(1), 100–125 (2014)
7. Castro, S., Ariel, W., Gómez, C., Danilo, Ó., Franco, O., Fernanda, L.: Selección de proveedoreS: una aproximación al estado del arte. no. Castro, S., Ariel, W., Gómez, C., Danilo, Ó., Franco, O., Fernanda, L. (2009). http://www.redalyc.org/articulo.oa?id=20511730008

8. Yadav, V., Sharma, M.K.: An application of hybrid data envelopment analytical hierarchy process approach for supplier selection. J. Enterp. Inf. Manag. **28**(2), 218–242 (2015)
9. Vírseda, L.: Revisión de los métodos, modelos y herramientas existentes para la selección de proveedores, pp. 1–11 (2011)
10. Kumar, D., Garg, C.P.: Evaluating sustainable supply chain indicators using fuzzy AHP: case of Indian automotive industry. Benchmarking **24**(6), 1742–1766 (2017)
11. Gil, M.: La Selección De Proveedores Elementos Clave En La Gestion De Aprovisionamientos, p. 63 (2018)
12. Shahgholian, K., Shahraki, A., Vaezi, Z.: Multi-Criteria Group Decision Making Method Based on, Management, no. ICM, pp. 461–471 (2011)
13. Lammi, H.: Supplier Evaluation and Selection Process, Helsinki Metropolia University of Applied Sciences (2011)
14. de Boer, L., Labro, E., Morlacchi, P.: A review of methods supporting supplier selection. Archit. Des. **80**(3), 66–73 (2001)
15. Castorena, O.H.: Proveedores y modelos de gestión en la cadena de suministro: Pymes manufactureras de Aguascalientes (México). Rev. Faccea **7**(1), 21–28 (2017)
16. Molamohamadi, Z., Ismail, N., Leman, Z., Zulkifli, N.: Supplier selection in a sustainable supply chain. J. Adv. Manag. Sci. **1**(3), 278–281 (2013)
17. Saaty, T.L., Sodenkamp, M.: The analytic hierarchy and analytic network measurement processes: the measurement of intangibles. Eur. J. PURE Appl. Math. **1**(1), 91–166 (2017)
18. Perçin, S.: An application of the integrated AHP-PGP model in supplier selection. Meas. Bus. Excell. **10**(4), 34–49 (2006)
19. Duica, M.C., Florea, N.V., Duica, A.: Selecting the right suppliers in procurement process along supply chain-a mathematical modeling approach. Valahian J. Econ. Stud. **9**(1), 47–58 (2018)
20. Lewis, C.: Linear Programming: Theory and Applications, Whitman Coll. Math. Dep. (2008)
21. Florez, L.A.P., Rodriguez-Rojas, Y.L.: Procedimiento de Evaluación y Selección de Proveedores Basado en el Proceso de Análisis Jerárquico y en un Modelo de Programación Lineal Entera Mixta. Ingeniería **23**(3), 230–251 (2018)
22. Hernadez-Ramirez, D., Bluhm-Gutierez, J., Valle-Rodriguez, S.: Conceptos Básicos De Programación Lineal Y Aplicación En El Manejo De Recursos Naturales. Ambient. y Sostenibilidad, no. February, p. 97 (2017)
23. Ter Chang, C.: Revised multi-choice goal programming. Appl. Math. Model. **32**(12), 2587–2595 (2008)
24. Azmi, R., Tamiz, M.: A Review of Goal Programming, no. September (2014)
25. Fullana, C., Urquia, E.: Los modelos de simulacion una herramienta multidiciplinar en investigacion. J. Chem. Inf. Model **32**, 1689–1699 (2009)
26. Salmasnia, A., Daliri, H., Ghorbanian, A., Mokhtari, H.: A statistical analysis and simulation based approach to an uncertain supplier selection problem with discount option. Int. J. Syst. Assur. Eng. Manag. **9**(6), 1250–1259 (2018)
27. Azadeh, A., Zarrin, M., Salehi, N.: Supplier selection in closed loop supply chain by an integrated simulation-Taguchi-DEA approach. J. Enterp. Inf. Manag. **29**(3), 302–326 (2016)
28. Abdullah, L., Chan, W., Afshari, A.: Application of PROMETHEE method for green supplier selection: a comparative result based on preference functions. J. Ind. Eng. Int. **15**(2), 271–285 (2019)
29. Gul, M., Celik, E., Gumus, A.T., Guneri, A.F.: A fuzzy logic based PROMETHEE method for material selection problems. Beni-Suef Univ. J. Basic Appl. Sci. **7**(1), 68–79 (2018)
30. Behzadian, M., Kazemzadeh, R.B., Albadvi, A., Aghdasi, M.: PROMETHEE: a comprehensive literature review on methodologies and applications. Eur. J. Oper. Res. **200**(1), 198–215 (2010)

31. Che, Z.H., Wang, H.S.: A hybrid approach for supplier cluster analysis. Comput. Math. with Appl. **59**(2), 745–763 (2010)
32. De La Hoz, E., Polo, L.L.: Aplicación de Técnicas de Análisis de Conglomerados y Redes Neuronales Artificiales en la Evaluación del Potencial Exportador de una Empresa. Inf. Tecnol. **28**(4), 67–74 (2017)
33. Matich, D.J.: Redes Neuronales: Conceptos Básicos y Aplicaciones. Historia Santiago, p. 55 (2001)
34. Chen, C.T., Lin, C.T., Huang, S.F.: A fuzzy approach for supplier evaluation and selection in supply chain management. Int. J. Prod. Econ. **102**(2), 289–301 (2006)
35. Yeung, J.F.Y., Chan, A.P.C., Chan, D.W.M.: Fuzzy set theory approach for measuring the performance of relationship-based construction projects in Australia. J. Manag. Eng. **28**(2), 181–192 (2012)
36. Tolun, M.R., Oztoprak, K.: Expert Systems. Handb. Chemoinformatics **3**, 1281–1294 (2008)
37. Giraldo, O.G.: Guía ejecutiva para el diseño y aplicación del método Delphi en la Prospectiva Laboral Cualitativa, ResearchGate, no. December 2013, pp. 0–28 (2013)
38. Abdi, H.: Kendall rank correlation coefficient, Concise Encycl. Stat., pp. 278–281 (2008)
39. Gavin, H.P.: The Levenburg-Marqurdt Algorithm For Nonlinear Least Squares Curve-Fitting Problems, Duke Univ., pp. 1–19 (2019)

Feasibility Analysis of a Supply Chain for Castor Oil Biodiesel Distribution in Central Mexico

Marcelo Galas-Taboada(✉) (iD)

Universidad Anáhuac México, Naucalpan de Juárez,, Mexico
marcelo.galas@anahuac.mx

Abstract. The aim of this paper is to analyze the feasibility of establishing a supply chain for castor oil biodiesel distribution in Central Mexico, based on the distribution of land with the highest castor oil seed yield potential. The supply chain analysis is focused on meeting the biodiesel demand for the region, assuming a B20 mix usage, from the proposed plantation sites to refineries and gas stations, using Network Optimization, and defining the required biodiesel production increase to achieve this.

Keywords: Supply chain · Biofuel · Biodiesel · Castor oil · Mexico · Dynamic systems · Optimization

1 Introduction

Currently, Mexico imports around 262 thousand barrels of diesel daily, which represent approximately 66.8% of the 392 thousand daily barrels that conform the average national demand. This means that only 130 thousand daily barrels of diesel are produced locally [1].

The current government campaigned with an agenda highly focused on sustainability and clean energies, however, the actual policies are oriented towards the exploration and exploitation of oil fields, together with investments in PEMEX, Mexico's state-owned oil company [2]. These policies seek to reduce Mexico's reliance on oil products imports, like gasoline and diesel.

Considering this objective, the production of biodiesel is presented as a sustainable aid to meet the diesel demand, with the added benefit of supporting the development of the agricultural sector.

In previous studies, it has been presented that the mass production of biodiesel based on commercially cultivated edible plants is not considered economically feasible given the shortage of food it would trigger with a subsequent rise of food prices. Taking this into account, other plants that meet the requirements must be considered as sources, as long as they do not cannibalize or endanger current food production capabilities. One such plant is the castor oil plant (Ricinus communis), which has a relatively high yield of biodiesel and whose byproducts can be used to create compost [3].

© ICST Institute for Computer Sciences, Social Informatics and Telecommunications Engineering 2021
Published by Springer Nature Switzerland AG 2021. All Rights Reserved
J. A. Marmolejo-Saucedo et al. (Eds.): COMPSE 2020, LNICST 359, pp. 86–98, 2021.
https://doi.org/10.1007/978-3-030-69839-3_6

Research into biofuels as an alternative to traditional fossil fuels is not new. There are several studies, from the private as well as public sectors, that analyze the issue from an energy potential point of view [4], as well as the production processes based on used vegetable oils [5] and the production costs [6].

There are studies that analyze the supply and demand of gasoline in Mexico, like *"The demand for gasoline in Mexico: Effects and alternatives considering climate change"* ("La demanda de gasolinas en México: Efectos y alternativas ante el cambio climático") by Reyes, Escalante and Matas or *"Demand for gasoline and heterogeneity in household income in Mexico"* ("Demanda de gasolina y la heterogeneidad en los ingresos de los hogares en México") by Sanchez, Islas and Sheinbaum.

Some other studies have focused on biodiesel and biofuels, such as *"Study on the Feasibility of the Use of Biodiesel in the Public Transport System of the Metropolitan Area of Guadalajara"* ("Estudio sobre la Viabilidad de la Utilización de Biodiesel en el Servicio Público de Transporte Colectivo del Área Metropolitana de Guadalajara") from 2014 by Alcocer and Uriarte, which focused on the feasibility of using palm oil biodiesel for the public transport system of Guadalajara. There is also a study from 2017, *"Analysis of the supply chains of bioethanol and biodiesel in Mexico: Case studies"* ("Análisis de las cadenas de suministro de bioetanol y biodiésel en México: Estudios de caso"), which focuses on the current production of bioethanol and biodiesel in Mexico, including a section on the production of biodiesel based on castor oil.

However, there are few studies that analyze the risks and performance of supply chains, and their technical feasibility, specially focused on the current socio-economic environment in Mexico. These studies would help promote the use of renewable energy sources in Mexico in a practical, sustainable, and responsible way.

2   Castor Oil

2.1   Castor Oil Production in Mexico

During the second semester of 2010, the National Institute for Forestry, Agricultural and Fishing Research (INIFAP, for its initials in Spanish, Instituto Nacional de Investigaciones Forestales, Agricolas y Pecuaria), concluded the project *"Study of Raw Materials for obtaining Biofuels in Mexico"* ("Estudio de Insumos para la Obtención de Biocombustibles en México") where they were able to obtain the following information: identification of the genetic potential for the creation of varieties with outstanding agro-industrial characteristics in pine nut (Jatropha curcas), castor (Ricinus communis) and sweet sorghum (Sorghum bicolor), and identification of the agroecological conditions for the cultivation of the Mexican pine nut, castor, sweet sorghum and beet (Beta vulgaris) [7].

Castor oil seed sales slumped for a time, when each kilogram of ground seed went for $3.00MXN in Oaxaca, for example. However, in recent years, it's price has gone up following the discovery of different applications for castor oil, to a point where it has become more profitable for some farmers to cultivate castor plants, at $8.00MXN per kilo, rather than their traditional crops of tomato, at $2.00MXN per kilo [8]. In some other instances, farmers grow castor plants as a side crop, for additional income, given that it can be grown alongside maize and beans [9, 10] (Table 1).

Table 1. Unit nomenclature used in the Mexican energy sector

Volume (liquids)	
Unit	Description
b	barrels
bd	barrels per day
Mb	thousands of barrels
Mbd	thousands of barrels per day
MMb	millions of barrels
MMbd	millions of barrels per day
m^3	cubic meters
m^3d	cubic meters per day
Mm^3	thousands of cubic meters
Mm^3d	thousands of cubic meters per day
MMm^3	millions of cubic meters
l	liters
gal	gallons

2.2 National Diesel Supply in Mexico

Between December 2018 and December 2019 (Fig. 1), the daily national average supply of diesel was 392 thousand barrels, of which, on average, 264 thousand barrels were imported daily, an equivalent of 67.35% of the total daily supply, leaving 32.65% to national diesel production [1].

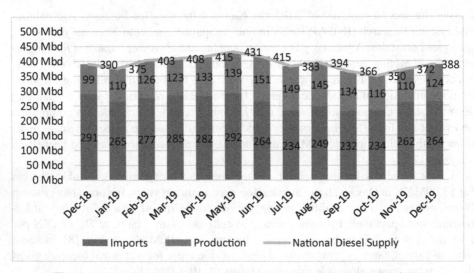

Fig. 1. National diesel supply, December 2018 to December 2019 (Mbd) [1]

3   Supply Chain Model Analysis

To evaluate different supply chain models based on meeting the demand of diesel and minimizing transportation costs, the selected analysis method is Network Optimization using AnyLogistix [11], a software tool for designing supply chains and managing them with a digital twin, which integrates supply chain design, optimization, and simulation with operations data.

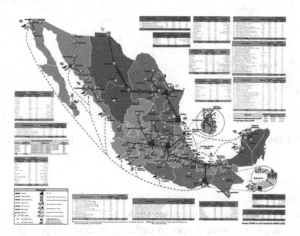

Fig. 2. National petroleum infrastructure [12]

Based on the production model presented in *"Biodiesel supply chain analysis in Mexico: case studies regarding biodiesel and castor oil plants as an alternative to imported diesel"* [3], in order to proceed with the analysis, the following initial assumptions were made:

- The creation of castor cultivation areas to meet the demand in biodiesel production must be considered.
- The storage and distribution centers (TARs for its initials in Spanish, Terminales de Almacenamiento y Reparto) of the national petroleum infrastructure (Fig. 2) will be used for storage, mixing at B20 and distribution of biodiesel.
- The transport of castor and biodiesel will be carried out using 31,000 kg tank trucks
- Biodiesel reserves, defined in the production model, will be distributed among the different TARs considered in the supply chain.

3.1   Castor Production Distribution

Because there is no access to the original data from which the map of suitable regions for the cultivation of castor (Fig. 3) was drawn, and their calculated yields, to carry out the distribution of the production capacity, a histogram analysis of the map was made in order to estimate this items. The regions considered for this analysis were Cerritos, in San Luis Potosí, and Tierra Blanca, in Veracruz. The yields used for the analysis were 850 kg/ha, for the light green/yellow areas, and 1.35 t/ha, for the dark green areas.

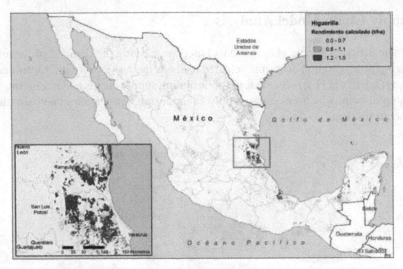

Fig. 3. Suitable regions for the cultivation of castor [13] (Color figure online)

Cerritos, San Luis Potosí

Based on the image for the region of Cerritos in San Luis Potosí (Fig. 4), which presents the largest concentration of soil with high yield of castor production, the histogram analysis is done by applying color filters in order to isolate the pixels corresponding to each yield level.

$$\frac{100 \text{ km}}{30 \text{ px}} * 197 \text{ px} = 656.67 \text{ km} \tag{1}$$

$$\frac{100 \text{ km}}{30 \text{ px}} * 157 \text{ px} = 523.33 \text{ km} \tag{2}$$

$$656.67 \text{ km} * 523.33 \text{ km} = 343,655.56 \text{ km}^2 = 34,365,555.56 \text{ ha} \tag{3}$$

Considering that the map scale shown in the image indicates there are 100 km per each 30 px, and that the image measure 197 px by 157 px, the surface presented in the map is approximately 34.365 million hectares.

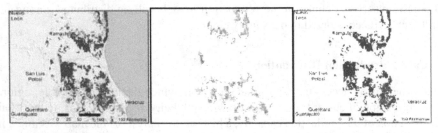

Fig. 4. Histogram analysis for Cerritos, San Luis Potosí – (own elaboration)

After applying the color filters, 13.72% of the image corresponds to high yield areas and 5.48% to medium/low yield areas.

$$13.72\% * 34,365,555.56 \text{ ha} = 4,714,954.22 \text{ ha} \tag{4}$$

$$5.48\% * 34,365,555.56 \text{ ha} = 1,883,232.44 \text{ ha} \tag{5}$$

This equals to around 4.714 million hectares of high yield soil and 1.883 million hectares of medium/low yield soil, which in total represents around 66% of the total national castor production capacity [14].

Considering a yield of 1.35 t/ha, for the high yield areas, and 0.85 t/ha, for medium/low yield areas, the amount of castor produced in the area can be calculated.

$$1.35\frac{t}{ha} * 4,714,954.22 \text{ ha} = 6,365,188.20 \text{ t} \tag{6}$$

$$0.85\frac{t}{ha} * 1,883,232.44 \text{ ha} = 4,600,747.58 \text{ t} \tag{7}$$

These calculations show that the region of Cerritos can produced around 10.966 million tons of castor per harvest.

Tierra Blanca, Veracruz
The second largest concentration of high yield castor production potential is in Tierra Blanca in Veracruz (Fig. 5), which is selected as the second region for the analysis.

$$\frac{195 \text{ km}}{31 \text{ px}} * 78 \text{ px} = 490.65 \text{ km} \tag{8}$$

$$\frac{195 \text{ km}}{31 \text{ px}} * 62 \text{ px} = 390 \text{ km} \tag{9}$$

$$490.65 \text{ km} * 390 \text{ km} = 191,351.6129 \text{ km}^2 = 19,135,161.29 \text{ ha} \tag{10}$$

Taking the border with Guatemala as a reference, the scale used on the map is 195 km for each 31 px, and the image measure 78 px by 62 px, which amounts to an approximate area of 19.135 million hectares.

After applying the color filters, the area of high yield equates to around 1.2% of the image and 5.96% correspond to medium/low yield soil.

$$1.2\% * 19,135,161.29 \text{ ha} = 229,621.94 \text{ ha} \tag{11}$$

Fig. 5. Histogram analysis for Tierra Blanca, Veracruz – (own elaboration)

$$5.96\% * 19,135,161.29 \text{ ha} = 1,140,455,61 \text{ ha} \qquad (12)$$

Considering the area covered by the image, the percentages represent around 229,621 ha of high yield soil and 1.140 million hectares of medium/low yield soil, around 13.69% of the total national castor production capacity [14].

Considering a yield of 1.35 t/ha, for the high yield areas, and 0.85 t/ha, for medium/low yield areas, the amount of castor produced in the area can be calculated.

$$1.35\frac{t}{ha} * 229,621.94 \text{ ha} = 309,989.61 \text{ t} \qquad (13)$$

$$0.85\frac{t}{ha} * 1,140,455,61 \text{ ha} = 969,387.27 \text{ t} \qquad (14)$$

Tierra Blanca can produce around 1.279 million tons of castor per harvest.

Ejido Yogana, Oaxaca
Given that there already exists a biodiesel refinery in Oaxaca, with a production capacity of 3 million litres of biodiesel per month, and that it acquires its castor from the Ejido Yogana, it was included in the model and its production surface estimated, considering a yield of 0.85 t/ha.

$$3,000,000 \, {}^{l\,(cbd)}\!/_{mes} * \frac{1\,mes}{30\,dias} * 180\frac{dias}{cosecha} = 18,000,000 \, {}^{l(cbd)}\!/_{cosecha} \qquad (15)$$

$$\frac{18,000,000 \, {}^{l(cbd)}\!/_{cosecha}}{232.05 \, {}^{l(cbd)}\!/_{ha}} = 77,569.49 \, ha/cosecha \approx 77,570 \, ha/cosecha \qquad (16)$$

Considering this, the Ejido Yogana has around 77,570 ha of castor per harvest.

3.2 Demand Distribution Within Central Mexico

There are 2,964 service stations in Central Mexico, according to the Listing of Service Stations of 2017 [15], distributed among the 7 states that conform the region. The states considered for the region are the following:

- Hidalgo
- Mexico City
- Morelos
- Puebla
- Queretaro
- State of Mexico
- Tlaxcala

Given the limitations of the educational license of AnyLogistix, which restricts the maximum number of customers to 100, an adjustment was made by calculating the percentage of service stations each state has, in relation to the total number of stations in the region, and a random selection was made based on this distribution (Table 2).

Table 2. Service stations in Central Mexico

States	Number of stations	Percentage	Sample size
Hidalgo	302	10%	10
Mexico City	376	13%	13
Morelos	172	6%	6
Puebla	576	19%	19
Queretaro	314	11%	11
State of Mexico	1,103	37%	37
Tlaxcala	121	4%	4
Total	2,964	100%	100

As the scope of this study is the analysis of the supply chain for the entire demand of castor biodiesel in a B20 mixture for Central Mexico, the total demand of each state was distributed among the number service stations that were taken as sample of each one in relation to the percentage they represent within the region (Table 3). For example, each one of the 10 stations selected to represent the state of Hidalgo, which has a daily demand of 1,799.67 barrels, is modeled as having a daily demand of 179.97 barrels.

Table 3. Daily demand per sampled station

States	Sampled service stations	Daily biodiesel consumption by state (barrels)	Daily biodiesel consumption by station (barrels)
Hidalgo	10	1,799.67	179.97
Mexico City	13	2,240.65	172.36
Morelos	6	1,024.98	170.83
Puebla	19	3,432.49	180.66
Queretaro	11	1,871.18	170.11
State of Mexico	37	6,572.98	177.65
Tlaxcala	4	721.06	180.27

3.3 Simulation and Analysis of the Supply Chain for Central Mexico

As was mentioned previously, this study will be using the existing TARs from the national petroleum infrastructure for the storage and distribution of biodiesel between the refineries and the service stations.

Given the analysis was done using an academic license of AnyLogistix, only 7 TARs in Central Mexico were selected and the other 3 available slots were used for the 3 refineries considered in this model (Fig. 6).

Two of these refineries are already in operation: Dertek, in the State of Mexico, with a monthly production capacity of 2,000,000 L of biodiesel, and Ricinomex, in Oaxaca, with a monthly production capacity of 3,000,000 L of biodiesel.

The third refinery is configured as a virtual source of biodiesel, in Poza Rica, which will help cover any deficit of biodiesel and will help to determine the amount of additional production of biodiesel required to fulfill the entire demand of Central Mexico.

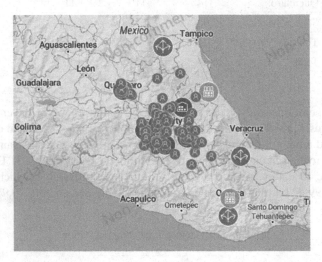

Fig. 6. Distribution of each member of the supply chain

To align the supply chain model to the production model, the supply chain simulation was broken up into blocks of 15 days with a maximum duration of 600 days (Table 4).

During the first 225 days, according to the production model, there is no consumption of biodiesel as production starts and stocks are created. Given this, the demand coefficient for these periods is set to zero.

Following these 225 days, the consumption start ramping up during the next 180 days until reaching the full biodiesel requirement for the region. This maximum consumption is represented in the demand coefficient as 1, which will be maintained until the end of the simulation, on day 600.

As the transportation medium for the raw materials and biodiesel, 31,000 kg tank trucks are being used at a cost of $1.08MXN per ton per kilometer [16], to establish the distribution routes and costs.

Using these parameters and restrictions, the network optimization was done to generate the supply chain represented in the following figures.

As seen on Fig. 7 and Fig. 8, out of the three proposed castor cultivation areas only two are used, Cerritos, in San Luis Potosi and Yogana, in Oaxaca.

The model considers the use of the three refineries, considering that the third refinery, the virtual one in Poza Rica, must produce around 33.4 million of liters each month,

Table 4. Simulation periods and demand coefficient

Period	Start date	End date	Demand coefficient
S1-S15	2020–01-01	2020–08-12	0
C1	2020–08-13	2020–08-27	0.077
C2	2020–08-28	2020–09-11	0.154
C3	2020–09-12	2020–09-26	0.231
C4	2020–09-27	2020–10-11	0.308
C5	2020–10-12	2020–10-26	0.385
C6	2020–10-27	2020–11-10	0.462
C7	2020–11-11	2020–11-25	0.538
C8	2020–11-26	2020–12-10	0.615
C9	2020–12-11	2020–12-25	0.692
C10	2020–12-26	2021–01-09	0.769
C11	2021–01-10	2021–01-24	0.846
C12	2021–01-25	2021–02-08	0.923
C13–C25	2021–02-09	2021–08-22	1

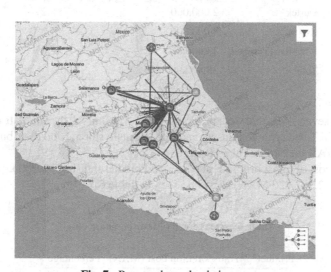

Fig. 7. Proposed supply chain map

approximately 87% of the total production, in order to fulfill the entire castor biodiesel demand (Table 5). This means that, to fulfill the production requirement, it is necessary to consider the construction of at least 12 refineries with the same capacity as Ricinomex.

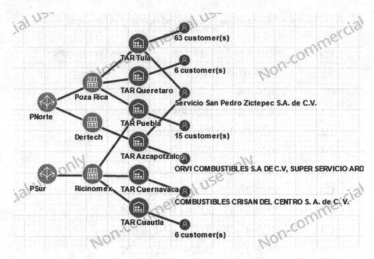

Fig. 8. Proposed supply chain structure

Table 5. Biodiesel production distribution

Refinery	Monthly Production (liters)	Percentage
Dertek	2,000,000	5.2%
Ricinomex	3,000,000	7.8%
Poza Rica *(virtual)*	33,400,000	87.0%
Total	38,400,000	100%

Out of the seven TARs that were programmed into the model, the simulation considers that the TAR in Toluca can go unused, and that the main storage and distribution will be done via the TAR located in Tula, Hidalgo.

The total cost of transportation, of castor and biodiesel, using 31,000 kg tank trunks was $4,367,022,707.026 MXN, as can be seen in Table 6.

Table 6. Breakdown of transportation cost

Product	Transportation cost (MXN)	Percentage
Castor	$3,575,808,800.254	82%
Biodiesel	$791,213,906.772	18%
TOTAL	$4,367,022,707.026	100%

4 Conclusions

Using a Network Optimization analysis, the results of the simulation of the supply chain model show that it is technically feasible to establish a supply chain that can completely meet the demand of castor biodiesel for Central Mexico, using a B20 mix. This is done using 6 TARs, 3 refineries and 2 cultivation areas.

As the simulation showed, there are enough lands with the potential to produce castor to meet the demand of castor biodiesel based on a B20 mix for Central Mexico, without exhausting them. This could potentially allow other regions of the country to take advantage of castor biodiesel to transition towards more sustainable and cleaner sources of energy.

Even though technically feasible, and considering that the virtual refinery produced the same amount of biodiesel as 12 refineries the size of Ricinomex, it would require an important investment to build the required refineries and establish the castor cultivation regions required to meet the demand of biodiesel.

A future study, using a commercial license of AnyLogistix, could use the supply chain model presented here and expand upon it, considering the entire universe of service stations and TARs that exist for Central Mexico, as well as the production capacity of each castor cultivation region, the storage capacities of each TAR, as well as the evaluation of possible risks.

Refining biodiesel from other types of raw materials, like used oils, also show great promise, however they face similar obstacles as castor biodiesel; mainly the logistics of collecting and transporting the raw materials to the refineries [17], as well as the policies toward renewable energy sources established by the current government in Mexico.

References

1. Secretaria de Energia. Prontuario estadístico de petrolíferos (2019)
2. Malkin, E.: López Obrador apuesta por la industria energética, pero Pemex está en crisis – Español. New York Times (2019)
3. Galas-Taboada, M., Aguirre-Macías, Y.P., López-Romero, Z.: Bioethanol and biodiesel supply chain analysis in mexico: case studies regarding biodiesel and castor oil plants. In: Vasant, P., Zelinka, I., Weber, G.-W. (eds.) ICO 2019. AISC, vol. 1072, pp. 531–540. Springer, Cham (2020). https://doi.org/10.1007/978-3-030-33585-4_52
4. Secretaria de Agricultura, Ganaderia, Desarrollo Rural P y A Bioenergéticos: higuerilla, jatropha curcas, sorgo dulce. Planeación agrícola Nac 2017–2030 (2017)
5. Gaurav, A., Ng, F.T.T., Rempel, G.L.: A new green process for biodiesel production from waste oils via catalytic distillation using a solid acid catalyst – Modeling, economic and environmental analysis. Green Energy Environ. 1, 62–74 (2016). https://doi.org/10.1016/j.gee.2016.05.003
6. Haas, M.J., McAloon, A.J., Yee, W.C., Foglia, T.A.: A process model to estimate biodiesel production costs. Bioresour. Technol. 97, 671–678 (2006). https://doi.org/10.1016/J.BIORTECH.2005.03.039
7. INIFAP Informe de autoevaluación de Director General del INIFAP correspondiente al ejercicio (2010)
8. Altamirano, N.: Higuerilla devuelve esperanza a mujeres de Yogana, Oaxaca (2018)

9. Ruiz, H.A., Martínez, A., Vermerris, W.: Bioenergy potential, energy crops, and biofuel production in Mexico. BioEnergy Res. **9**(4), 981–984 (2016). https://doi.org/10.1007/s12 155-016-9802-7

10. Sheinbaum, C., Balam, M.V., Robles, G., et al.: Biodiesel from waste cooking oil in Mexico City. Waste Manag. Res. **33**, 730–739 (2015). https://doi.org/10.1177/0734242X15590471

11. anyLogistix: Supply Chain Optimization, Simulation & Design Software Tools. https://www. anylogistix.com/

12. Secretaria de Energia Infraestructura Nacional de Petrolíferos (2018)

13. Riegelhaupt, E., Odenthal, J., Janeiro, L.: Diagnóstico de la situación actual del biodiésel en México y escenarios para su aprovechamiento. ECOFYS (2016)

14. Rico Ponce, H.R., Tapia Vargas, L.M., Teniente Oviedo, R., et al.: Guía para Cultivar Higuerilla (Ricinus communis L.) en Michoacán (2011)

15. CRE Estaciones de Servicio (Gasolineras) y Precios finales de Gasolina y Diesel (2017). https://datos.gob.mx/busca/dataset/estaciones-de-servicio-gasolineras-y-precios-fin ales-de-gasolina-y-diesel

16. Herrera, E.: Transportar gasolina en México es más caro. Milenio (2020)

17. Sheinbam-Pardo, C., Calderon-Irazoque, A., Ramirez-Suarez, M.: Potential of biodiesel from waste cooking oil in Mexico. Biomass Bioenerg. **56**, 230–238 (2013)

Automation of Storage and Distribution Terminals: The Case of Logistics Operators

Jania Saucedo Martinez[1], Carlos Regalao Noriega[2(✉)], and Luis Ortiz Ospino[2]

[1] Facultad de Ingenieria Mecanica y Electrica, Universidad Autonoma de Nuevo Leon,
Ciudad Universitaria, San Nicolas de los Garza, Nuevo Leon, Mexico
jania.saucedomrt@uanl.edu.mx
[2] Facultad de Ingenierias, Universidad Simon Bolivar, Barranquilla, Atlantico, Colombia
{crega-lao,lortiz27}@unisimonbolivar.edu.co

Abstract. Thinking about the logistics of an organization means grouping together all the processes of loading, routing, and distribution of the finished product to the end customer. The project proposes to study the automation of storage and distribution terminals: The case of the logistic operators of the department of Atlantico for the improvement of the decision making in the distribution activities in relation to the logistic operators of the department of Atlantico - Colombia for the improvement of the business effectiveness. Therefore, in the present investigation, a research is made, which uses a defined methodology and which leads to observe some results and conclusions framed in the categories: Intralogistics, Automation, Technologies 4.0, Business efficiency, which seeks to validate through the statistical application the importance of these as a resource to the insufficiencies that are represented in the environment of the logistics operators of the Department of Atlantico.

Keywords: Intralogistics · Automation · Technologies 4.0 · Business efficiency

1 Introduction

Humanity, as recorded in our history, has needed products in its living, which are generally not accessible, nor are they found or produced in the place of origin or in the place you want to consume. Foods and other essential products of coexistence are widely dispersed and only accessible in abundance at specific times and places. The ancient civilizations managed to consume only the most immediate food to their environment, for the time still did not have transportation and methods of In the case of modern storage, the movement of food or goods was limited to the capacity that a group of people could mobilize personally, and therefore, the storage of perishable food was only available for a short period time, forcing individuals to settle close to the sources of production in order to use the food and goods that could be produced in the environment or granted by nature. One can still see striking models of developing nations in Asia, South America, Australia, and Africa, where a group of their inhabitants lives in small, self-sufficient

© ICST Institute for Computer Sciences, Social Informatics and Telecommunications Engineering 2021
Published by Springer Nature Switzerland AG 2021. All Rights Reserved
J. A. Marmolejo-Saucedo et al. (Eds.): COMPSE 2020, LNICST 359, pp. 99–114, 2021.
https://doi.org/10.1007/978-3-030-69839-3_7

villages, where a large proportion of the goods needed by the people are produced or purchased in the immediate vicinity. By the above, it is evident that logistics is vital for the daily development of an individual or a community, which is why companies today are exploring various options in the area of logistics and supply chain management as a representation of a context of multiple concepts, rules, and theories, from the most conservative disciplines of marketing, production, accounting, purchasing, and transportation, to the areas of applied mathematics, organizational behavior, and economics, to provide solutions to the consumption needs of human beings on a global scale, according to modern paradigms.

Therefore, the logistic activities that take place inside the cities are of great importance for the economic and social growth of the communities, in particular, the Logistics Operators and their supply chain. For the specific case of the Colombian Caribbean region, specifically in the Department of Atlantico and in its capital city, Barranquilla, which is the object of this research project, where organizations respond to the continuous operation of the different economic and industrialized movements. Therefore, adopting the definition of the supply chain as: "The Supply Chain, or simply Supply Chain, is a chain of suppliers, factories, warehouses, distribution centers, and retailers through which raw materials are acquired, transformed and sent to the customer" [1]. The intralogistics processes of logistics operators account for almost 30% of the logistics costs of organizations in Colombia, which, according to the Colombian National Planning Department, represent approximately 15% of an organization's sales [2]. In Colombia, the intervention in logistics and especially the area of intralogistics continues in debt, and those modest processes within the organization, but of great organizational relevance increase the costs of all the products that must be transported on the domestic market [3]. Following Crespo [4] "The logistical cost in the country is several percentage points from the evidence of other nations in America and Europe. This shows that in comparison with the USA it represents only 8,7% of the sales achieved, in Europe, it increases to 11,9% and in Latin America, the estimate is around 14,7%".

Among the elements, the costs, in the intralogistics is a preponderant factor in all the economies of the world. In Colombia, we do not have the data on how much represents this value over the total of the logistic distribution and the supply chain, but for example for Brazil, it constitutes on average 28% of the costs, that is to say, that a good part of the value of a product towards the final consumer [5]. Therefore, in order to find tools that tend to improve decision-making that impact the indicators and in turn, the factors that determine the index of organizational efficiency in logistics operators. These requirements are delimited by three main scenarios: The First Scenario called Operational: The objective of this one focuses on the improvement of the processes in the intralogistic activities regarding the loading and unloading of the warehouse, emphasizing the point of view of the suppliers, to influence the synergy that must be developed as a pillar of the logistic operators and the performance of their human capital in the role of adaptation or non-adaptation of the new technologies in the framework of the industry 4.0. The second scenario described as Structural: It is defined as a valuable component for the execution of the activities of the logistics operators from the evaluation of the objectivity of the organization, according to the use of spaces for the intralogistic processes of raw materials and finished products. The third scenario is the Results: Which develops the items in the decision making process for the improvement of the organizational efficiency using the same based on the implementation of a simulation model via optimization, meeting the demands of the internal and external client of the logistics operators under study in this project. From the above, the problems presented by the organizations within their intralogistics processes are determined, defined in the aspects the non-existent value chain, unmanaged storage, low technological investment, lack of human talent, and the lack of cost vs. Income structure, which derives from aspects such as high costs in urban centers, increased lab our costs, low productivity, the non-adoption of new technologies and organizational efficiency rates below the region's standard, as shown in Fig. 1.

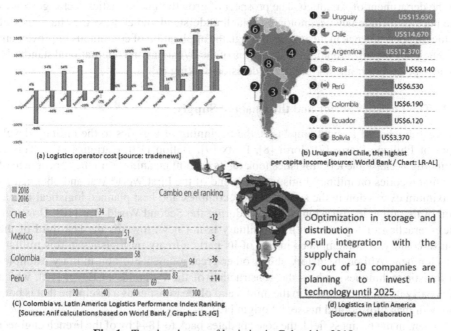

(a) Logistics operator cost [source: tradenews]

(b) Uruguay and Chile, the highest per capita income [source: World Bank / Chart: LR-AL]

(C) Colombia vs. Latin America Logistics Performance Index Ranking [Source: Anif calculations based on World Bank / Graphs: LR-JG]

(d) Logistics in Latin America [Source: Own elaboration]

Fig. 1. Trend and state of logistics in Colombia, 2018

1.1 Needs of Logistics Operators in the Caribbean Region

According to the proposed problem, the objective of this research is focused on: Improve the organizational efficiency index by implementing 4.0 technologies using simulation as a tool for decision making in the intralogistics processes of the Logistics Operators of the Atlantico department. As key points of this investigation, we will be looking to meet the following specific aspects: i) Performing a diagnosis of intralogistics processes and 4.0 technologies in the logistics operators of the Department of Atlantico. ii) Design the simulation model where the scenarios for the decision making on whether to implement industry 4.0 technologies in the intralogistic processes of logistics operators. iii) Evidencing by means of statistics the relevance of the object of study of the present project as a reference framework in the implementation of 4.0 technologies in intralogistic processes. iv) To evaluate the scenarios proposed for the improvement of intralogistic processes and the significant improvement of the organizational efficiency of the population studied.

This article establishes the premise that such a scenario assessment will provide greater certainty in decision-making for the implementation of 4.0 technologies in a general comparative framework of the organization's needs and will open the door to a global approach that contemplates the development, implementation and research in other industry sectors in their intralogistic processes. It is possible to measure the organizational efficiency indexes in the factors that impact the decision making, by means of the implementation of simulation in intralogistic processes of the logistic operators of the department of Atlantico. The prospect of growth in the logistics sector generates the need to include new technologies, which understand and address the challenges of achieving permanence in the market through the application of continuous improvement of efficiency organizational, from the vision of the dynamics and international standards, main aspects that frame an intelligent decision making [6].

1.2 The Logistics Sector and the Chain of Supply

A great number of authors emphasize the beginning of logistics to the military development Philippe-Pierre [7], Jordi [8], Roux [9], Ballou [10], Carranza [11]. This is primarily because the term logistics took on its current meaning from the appearance of the first theories on military logistics at the end of the First World War and obtained its maximum expression in the so-called most complex and best planned logistical operation of that time: the invasion of Europe during the Second World War [10]. However, the interaction of logistics with the military is not new; towards the last third of the fourth century, it contemplates in one of its parts a treaty on logistics in this military development. Although, history shows other great moments of non-military examples in logistic techniques such as the construction of the Pyramids of Egypt [12], which demystify its exclusive origin in the militia and place logistics as a discipline that is born the with man himself and his social origin [13].

Then, in the business field, the concept dates back to 1844 by of the French engineer Jules Dupuit who supported the idea of exchanging (Trade-off) a cost for other (transportation costs for storage costs) and the selection between land and water transport based on cost criteria [10]. The first documents dedicated to business logistics appeared in 1961 [14]. They define the benefits of organized logistics management. At the same time, Drucker [15], emphasized the concept of logistics as one of the last frontiers with real possibilities to improve business efficiency and described it as "the dark continent of the economy" [12]. The National Council of Physical Distribution Management (NCPDM), created in 1963, officially defined the concept of logistics as follows "A set of activities that are responsible for the efficient movement of finished products from the end of the production line to the consumer and that, in some cases, includes the movement of raw materials from the source to the line" [16]. Thus, even in these times, the definition of logistics was limited only to the activity of physical distribution. However, throughout the 1970s, special attention began to be paid to purchasing and handling of inputs at the beginning of the production chain. Consequently, the MRP (Materials Resource Planning) model was born as a solution to the problem of minimizing costs and providing some flexibility to the company, because the management and supply of inputs had been developed under the subordination to the function of the production process [17]. However, the management of the supply chain, in synthesis is defined as the planning, organization and control of the activities of the supply chain; defined in a wider way by the CSCMP: "The strategic and systematic combination in the competences of the traditional business and the tactics used inside the different companies of a supply chain, to improve the long term performance of the organizations individually as well as in the whole supply chain".

1.3 The Simulation in the Intralogistic Processes and Its Relation in the Industry 4.0

The continuous changes and advances in logistics and production systems make improvements and decision making necessary. Simulation is a good support tool for this type of action. Based on "what if" analysis, simulation allows us to reproduce processes and study their behavior, to analyze the impact of possible changes, or to compare different design alternatives without the high cost of full-scale experiments. Three basic components in the decision process that must be determined to formulate a simulation model, which are: i) The decision variables, ii) Problem constraints and, iii) Determine the objective function to be optimized.

Usually, the word simulation is related to computer tools such as video games or virtual reality, and in the case of the Air Force, to the word "war games" or "flight simulator". But in the design and optimization of logistics processes, simulation is defined as the process by which constructs, executes, and analyzes a process or case, following the variables and restrictions of real life. However, many models, due to their complexity, require time to design and execute them: also, the model validation process is usually complex as the system becomes more complex. The achievement of organizational efficiency must be referred to the corresponding business plan, which sets out the vision, mission, objectives, and corporate strategies based on a situational diagnosis. The use of management factors and indicators become the vital signs of the organization and are defined as useful tools in the procedure of making a decision, primarily when there are accurate data and enough time available to make the respective analysis. At its most basic level, analysis implies, fundamentally, looking for relationships between organized data, which can lead to: i) Identify correlations and cause-effect relationships between indicators, ii) Determining trends and building projections for an indicator and, iii) Carry out comparisons for the performance of an indicator.

Taking into account the above, it is necessary to establish evaluation methods that allow the capture of both quantitative and qualitative information [18], defines: "Logistics Performance Indicators as measures of quantifiable performance applied to logistics management that allow to evaluating the performance and the result in each process of reception, storage, inventories, dispatch, distribution, delivery, invoicing and information flow between the parts of the logistic chain. It is essential that every company develops skills around the management of logistics management indicators, to be able to use the resulting information on time manner".

1.4 Importance of Improving Business Efficiency

The organizations that are making their way into the third decade of the 21st century are self-directed in achieving and evidencing a higher performance in their processes, by controlling the negative impact that today generates the intralogistics within the supply chain and the adoption of technologies of the industry 4.0, which allows us to observe that organizations are in the development of adapting and structuring their processes to international requirements and standards. The collaborative integration of the supply chain is based on establishing multiple planning activities and defines the various information changes. Colombia, its departments and cities suffer from this scourge in intralogistics, especially the Caribbean Region which observe a significant impact on the levels of productivity and competitiveness concerning to other regions of the country and Latin America; the current administration of President Ivan Duque framed in the National Development Plan 2018–2022. The Future Belongs to All and the strategic work of the Department of Atlantico of Governor Elsa Noguera Atlantico is the people, added to the district strategic plans of the mayors of the cities of the department, include an item especially and of rigorous compliance for logistical. Studies conducted worldwide, according to Both of [19], determine that logistics costs as a percentage of GDP in Latin American and Caribbean countries are set to be between 50% and 100% higher than in the member countries of the Organization for Economic Cooperation and Development (OECD). In Colombia in particular, the lack of progress in road infrastructure has led to less efficient land-based freight transport, problems with port capacity and competition, and a small increase in other internal modes of transport such as rail (used only for coal transport) or river transport, which also harms on logistics operators. Likewise, The BDI [20], states that the sector of logistics operators presents a great opportunity for small businesses, considering that logistics management is part of the most strategic processes of organizations, where the costs that this generates represent 19% of the Gross Domestic Product (GDP) in Latin American countries like Colombia, justified mainly by the complexity of the customs processes among other factors. State, business and academia agree that technologies of industry 4.0 will play a decisive role in the efficiency levels at superlative degrees causing all organizations to establish a synopsis of continuous improvement, high productivity and competitiveness in their activities [20]. The growing business innovation in technological aspects emanating from industry 4.0 that we are experiencing today indicates that the organizations that adapt to these demands will be prepared to know, develop and apply the solutions that provide this technological boom, where simulation via optimization will be highly linked to decision-making in the operations and activities of the organizations, especially to the intralogistic aspects of the logistics operators. Accordingly, the Private Competitiveness Council (CPC) agreed with the World Bank's Logistics Performance Index for the period 2018–2019. In 2018 Colombia obtained the highest rating in its history in the logistics performance index, where it advanced 36 positions compared to 2016 (it went from 94th to 58th place) and today it is fifth in Latin America [21], as shown in Fig. 2. However, there are still challenges in: efficiency and effectiveness of customs, quality of infrastructure, competition and quality of logistics services [20]. Freight transport in the country concentrated in road mode, of the 2400 registered transport companies, around 2000 are informal and only 25% of drivers are formalized [20].

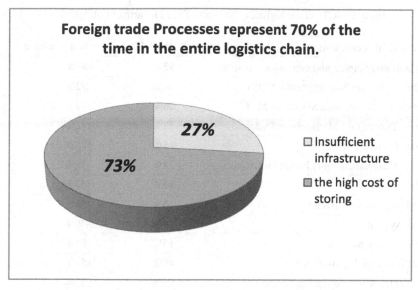

Fig. 2. Logistics Performance Index. Colombia and reference countries, 2018.

The result of the Logistics Performance Index Fig. 2 of the World Bank is ratified by the DNP national logistics survey, in which users of the in addition to insufficient infrastructure, logistics bottlenecks are caused by the high cost of storing, loading and unloading goods, inefficient information systems, inefficient procedures, lack of areas for loading and unloading goods, and a shortage of human capital and logistics areas, among other factors. The country, then, is not unaware of the existence of a higher level of competitiveness in the field. Therefore, one of the major advances the country's most important event was the preparation of the CONPES document [27], called the National Logistics Plan, which was approved in 2018 and established the policy guidelines, infrastructure needs and inclusion of 4.0 technologies, and financing for the development of actions to increase competitiveness through the adoption of better logistics practices. The development plan Atlantic Departmental Territorial Development Vision 2020: The route for development (2025) lays down the guidelines in which it should focus its efforts on the growth of competitiveness and economic strengthening. In the same way, the development plan of the current district administrations is articulated to the same guidelines [22]. Table 1 shows the current level of penetration of ICT applied to the logistics industry and in particular its availability in the country's logistics operators.

Table 1. ICTs in the logistics operators of the Department of Atlantico

ICTs in logistics operators	Available	Not available
Optimization, planning and control of transport	57%	43%
Distribution Center Management (WMS)	28%	72%
Distribution Management System (DMS)	28%	72%
Business Transaction Management/Orders	28%	72%
Integrated WMS TMS	15%	85%
Demand management and planning software	24%	76%
ERP Interfaces	33%	67%
Fleet Management Software	45%	55%
Barcode system	24%	76%
Radiofrequency System	15%	85%
System for Invoicing/Auditor's	49%	51%
Real-time tracking and tracing system	73%	27%
Internet access for the client	63%	37%
Electronic Data Interchange System (EDI)	24%	76%
Picking Optimization System	15%	85%

The results show a degree of use of ICTs that is not very high since according to the trends of the sector at an international level it would be desirable to have penetration levels above 80%, however, none of the categories of ICTs analyzed reach that level of availability. In this way, it can be seen that although Colombia has made progress in modernizing the provision of logistics operations services, especially in activities linked to intralogistics processes, where there are still lags in terms of infrastructure, and performance indicators.

2 Methodology

The project method is part of the Operations Management research line regarding the study of the thematic axis of supply chains from the perspective of intralogistics operations. From a process of direct observation and analysis to determine the factors that influence decision-making according to the scenarios in the implementation or not of 4.0 technologies in the case of logistics operators in the department of Atlantico. From the above, a three-phase research process is proposed:

i)   It begins with a general characterization of the companies studied taking as a reference to analysis of the vertical and horizontal integration systems within the framework of industry 4.0. This is a photograph of the current reality that is presented in the logistics operators according to the factors under study.

ii) Next, using the computer package and the use of the statistical tool, the possible scenarios are established for the factors under study in this project.

iii) It continues with establishing quantitatively which are the factors that allow the evaluation of the scenarios and the impact of implementing or not the technologies of Industry 4.0 and which significantly impact intralogistics processes in the search for improvement in organizational efficiency, through simulation via optimization evaluated in the computational tool.

2.1 General Characterization of the Company

This section consists of evaluating the entire system of operations of the logistic operators, for which the procedure defined by Perez [23] was used, in which three considerations stand out in the characterization process: integration On vertical, horizontal and, as the last point, the use of Industry 4.0 technologies, Table 2 describes them.

Table 2. Mapping the organizational structure

Consideration	Description
Vertical integration	It is based on the socio-technical system and the value creation modules
Horizontal integration	It is based on operations management requirements
Technologies 4.0	It contains the tools studied in the literature analysis

The mapping delimited in Table 2 allows us to know the organization in general, that is, it shows the outstanding elements and activities, deficient situations and critical points of the process, consequently the ordered form of the instrument used to characterize the logistic operators as a function of its vertical and horizontal integration systems within the framework of Industry 4.0 technologies. From the above, we can see in Fig. 3 the diagnostic result of the vertical and horizontal integration systems within the framework of the technologies of Industry 4.0, of the company which is the object of this research, which allows us to deduce the degree of absorption which is presented in the intralogistic activities of the logistics operators and to delimit the roadmap towards the continuous improvement of the indicators of organizational efficiency.

However, in the characteristics of horizontal integration, more work needs to be done. In this case, the diagnosis shows that the external perception shows 59% adaptability and the internal vision only reaches 53%, which generates interesting opportunities.

Vertical and horizontal integration systems in the framework of industry 4.0: Evaluation and development

General Information

Type of evaluation		Diagnosis	x	Responsible
		Follow up		Carlos Regalao Noriega

Evaluators			Name of the organization:				Logycem - Logística al Día
	Quantity		Size of the organization People- Income				Type of organization:
Position held: Customer	4		Micro	Small	Medium	Large	
Provider	4					x	Manufacturing x
Operational	2						Technologies
Director	1						Services

Diagnostic results

System evaluation

Vertical integration	65%	64%		Horizontal integration		59%	53%
			Dif				

Left	%	%	Dif	Right	Dif.	%	%
Human	63%	62%	-1%	**Supply**		64%	60%
Human Integration	59%	51%	-8%	Relationship Management	-5%	66%	61%
Administrative staff	63%	64%	1%	Information flow	-2%	60%	58%
Operational personnel	66%	70%	4%	Vendor evaluation	-7%	67%	61%
Organization	67%	68%		Comprehensive decisions	-2%	61%	59%
Development and interrelations	70%	72%	2%	**Planning and administration**		52%	47%
Information Management	63%	63%	0%	Administration	-6%	63%	57%
Team				Programming	-7%	41%	34%
Cyber-physical interaction	59%	58%	-1%	Simulation	-2%	53%	50%
Processes	64%	64%		**Customer Service**		60%	58%
Development of operations	57%	55%	-2%	Order Management	-1%	45%	44%
Lean Manufacturing	67%	70%	3%	Inventory Management	0%	63%	64%
Implementation of Core Tools	69%	67%	-1%	Warehouse Management	-5%	70%	64%
Product	67%	64%		Materials management	-5%	64%	59%
Research and Development	62%	59%	-2%	Transportation Management	-4%	59%	54%
Technology	60%	58%	-2%	Customer Service	-1%	61%	60%
Sustainability	79%	75%	-4%				

Tools 4.0			61%	59%		
Big data and analysis	61%	59%	3D manufacturing	63%	64%	
Autonomous robots	62%	61%	Augmented reality	53%	48%	
Simulation	54%	52%	The Cloud	61%	59%	Smooth perception (internal,
Integration systems	62%	60%	Advanced materials	79%	75%	
Industrial Internet of Things	61%	59%	Virtual Reality	62%	61%	External perception
Cybersecurity	60%	58%				Difference

* External perception is excluded from internal processes

Fig. 3. Vertical and horizontal integration systems in the framework of industry 4.0: Evaluation and development

2.2 Scenarios Understudy

There are different ways to approach the future, to foresee the needs of an organization and to strive for its continuous improvement; In the case of the present study, the methodological aim is to build scenarios through the implementation of simulation as a tool that allows analyzing the impact on the inclusion of the technologies of Industry

4.0 and defining implementation proposals for the analysis of the different options for solutions to the problem studied. To see Fig. 4.

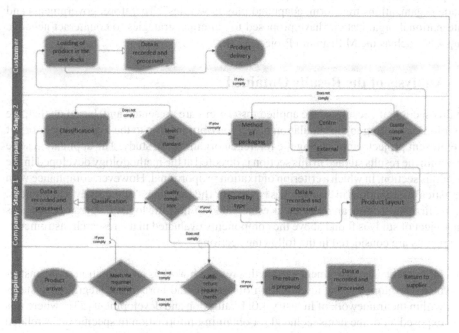

Fig. 4. Current scenario of the company understudy

In a warehouse, the main objective of the improvement is focused on the optimization of space and on providing means of handling loads normally at high heights and with medium volumes of work. While in a Distribution Center the optimization focuses on a rapid flow of materials and the optimization of labor, especially in Picking tasks.

Table 3. Optimization characteristics in the study setting

	Warehouse	Distribution center
Principal function	Storage management and inventory layout	Flow management products
"Cost driver" Principal	Space and facilities	Transport, Hand working
Order cycle	Months, weeks	Days, hours
Activities of value-added	Punctual, in rotation cyclical	They are an intrinsic part of process
Expeditions	On customer demand and Vendors	According to orders
Rotation of inventory	3, 6, 9, 12	12, 24, 48, 96, 120

The above is visualized and studied in the present scenario, where concepts of plant distribution, process optimization and reorganization of functions are involved to solve the problem. Thus, as Jung [24] put it, "the new world scenario of globalization has made organizations transform, adapt and play new roles". Therefore, governments and international organizations have proposed to generate strategies to counteract negative impacts, such as the Millennium Project, [25].

3   Analysis of the Results Obtained

In this section, the results of the applied instrument are presented and, based on that, the solutions according to the simulation model via optimization to the logistic operators of the present project, emphasizing the reference organization study. The application style to obtain the results studied in this section is directed at the methodology developed in the previous section, in which a criterion of fixation proportional. However, compliance with statistical assumptions in the analyzes is vital for the usefulness of the study's inferences. In the first subsection, an overview is established of how the logistic operator chosen as the object of study is found above the components evaluated in the research instruments, the results are considered in the following sections:

i)   Instrument: The instrument used in this research work is an adaptation of the instrument developed in the investigation of vertical and horizontal integration systems within the framework of Industry 4.0: Evaluation and development [23]:, where it is exposed all of the items included for obtaining information in specific areas related to vertical and horizontal integration systems, as well as the development and use of technology. It is the level at which an instrument produces consistent and coherent results [26]. Cronbach's alpha has been used in the research to measure internal consistency, locating the results from variances or through correlations between reagents, in this case, the following formula is used

$$\alpha = \left[\frac{k}{k-1}\right][1 - \sum_{i=1}^{k} \frac{S_i^2}{S_t^2}] \tag{1}$$

Where: k is the number of reagents.
Reliability testing is carried out through the supply of measurement instruments, to prove their effectiveness in the logistics operators' sector. To this end, an evaluation was carried out in which various organizations were included A total of 44 agents took part in a critical review of which the organization under study was selected as adopting the main characteristics and adaptable to other organizations in the sector. This test was carried out by mean of cronbach alpha resulting in $\alpha = 0.98$; It can be stated that the structure of the measuring instrument based on the reliability criterion is in the range of excellent.

ii)   Scenarios: Scenarios are defined as the events that can occur or dissipate in the possibility of applying or not applying the simulation model by means of optimization, the Flexsim software is applied as a simulation tool and develops the problem situation studied with its distinctive results which can be seen in Table 4, determined in the result of the analysis of the vertical and horizontal integration systems.

Table 4. Table of analysis of the projected scenarios

Factors	Indicators	Scenarios		
		Current	Different distribution or layout	Technology 4.0
Information management	Volume of purchases	32.12%	30.59%	34.55%
	Inventory time	28.56%	36.45%	50.61%
Strategic planning	Perfect delivery received	36.54%	30.29%	44.37%
	Inventory time	28.78%	50.18%	58.85%
	Types of transport	22.54%	82.62%	59.93%
	Punctuality of the offices	30.23%	42.51%	73.17%
Subcontracting	Perfect delivery received	8.71%	14.63%	44.77%
Business model	Certificate of suppliers	54.38%	74.48%	84.49%
Logistic barriers	Quality of infrastructure	64.81%	80.07%	90.45%
Cost	Order quality	70.23%	58.15%	68.38%
	Perfect delivery received	36.19%	30.74%	44.02%
	Inventory time	28.70%	36.52%	38.27%
Risk	Volume of purchases	22.76%	38.38%	28.68%
	Efficiency in the offices customs officers	82.94%	86.17%	84.48%
Distribution strategy	Types of transport	8.67%	6.05%	11.33%
	Punctuality of the offices	40.42%	30.72%	44.57%

i) Supplier aspect: This item defines the capabilities, relationship, communication and integration that the company under study has with organizations that provide you with the inputs for your operation.

ii) Organization aspect: It defines the aspects inherent to intralogistics within the company, synthesizes the object of study of this research project; it is defined as the item that contains the aspects of improvement in and adaptation of the different scenarios that can be designed.

iii) Customer aspect: It develops the dependent and independent variables according to the requirements of the product and the needs of the client; it allows the measurement of the organizational efficiency indicator and the parameters for it.

iv) Evaluation: It consists of the results of the tests of objectivity, validation and reliability of the simulation model. Table 4, presents the comparison of results between the Factors in accordance with the indicators that interact and how these vary according to the scenario in which they are used, with which we can determine that the inclusion of technologies of the industry 4.0.

The previous table shows the results obtained by simulating the established scenarios using the Flexsim tool and parameterized in the statistical and control assumptions in accordance with the results derived from the instrument applied in this research and the aspects developed with the applied diagnosis of the vertical and horizontal integration systems in the framework of industry 4.0.

v) Research Analysis: Shows the analysis of the organization object of study of the logistics operators of the department of the Atlantic pertaining to the results of the diagnosis, the analysis of the model of simulation and recommendations for its evolution to industry 4.0 technologies. It was also defined that the analysis factors are those identified as Information Management, Business Model and Logistic Barriers, the latter being the which benefits most from the adoption of 4.0 technologies in the intralogistics activities of logistics operators, and which represents an increase in infrastructure quality of 90.45%.

4 Conclusions and Discussions of Information Analysis

In this work, a quantitative research was carried out, framed in a positivist epistemological approach, that is, it is based on the analysis of real facts that are validated by experience, seeking to find the main factors that intervene in a simulation process through the optimization for the inclusion of technologies of the Industry 4.0 in the intralogistics activities, that allow to improve the organizational efficiency. The results of the research identify trends related to establishing that there is an association between the predominant factors and indicators in the logistics sector, specifically in the logistics operators, primarily in relation to the scenarios studied.

Consequently, it is necessary to build decision models that receive these results as input and provide solutions to intralogistic processes using Industry 4.0 technologies in strategic and operational spaces, not only for decision making but also to provide coordination mechanisms between the different variables involved in relation to the supply chain. In this sense, the literature proposes to explore relationship alternatives based on operating costs in intralogistics processes and the supply chain. The research carried out in the present study, as mentioned above, has determined that the logistics operators of the department of Atlantico object of study of this project, the factors that influence are the costs as a dependent variable, the Planning factors strategic and Subcontracting. For this reason, it is recommended to replicate the present research work and its methodology for the study of the sectors in which cargo loading and unloading tasks are carried out regarding various types of logistics, in order to identify opportunities for improvement. In the aspects studied in this project. In terms of the Business efficiency, the organizations under study have a dynamic system in the way that they operationalize their processes in relation to intralogistic processes. The need for flexibility in industry 4.0 technologies is prioritized in order to be more efficient, consistently impacting the costs of supply chain operations or activities in intralogistics of the logistic operators. The first reflection of the present study and of the logistics operating organizations is to consider the importance of assuming a commitment to the articulation of strategies that promote the reduction of costs in terms of the implementation of Industry 4.0 technologies in intralogistic processes, generate better mechanisms and contribute to improving decision-making. In other words, building a collaborative policy that allows working on the opportunity that intralogistics provides for the supply chain and the logistics operators sector. However, one must work on the simulation model optimization that addresses the right strategies for each of the actors and takes into account It takes into account the variables studied in the present project, the future windows of study and the complexities that may arise as the topic addressed is deepened. In another thematic line, it is highlighted that the government must seek a way to regulate the tax positions of the cities that make life in the department of Atlantico, because it has been found that the economic environment tends to vary according to the fleet of the company that circulates through cities of the metropolitan area from Barranquilla. For this reason, companies choose conservative investment strategies that slow down the expansion of businesses and it is necessary to establish for this study an analysis unit that guarantees the type of additional information that logistics operators require. For decision making and the continuous search for the improvement of organizational efficiency.

References

1. Lambert, D.M., Cooper, M.C., Pagh, J.D.: Supply chain management: implementation issues and research opportunities. Int. J. Logist. Manag. **9**(2), 1–20 (1998). https://doi.org/10.1108/09574099810805807
2. DIAN: Dirección de Impuestos y Aduanas Nacionales, 07 July 2018. https://www.dian.gov.co/. Accessed 23 Oct 2019
3. Silva, J.D.: Gestión de la cadena de suministro: una revisión desde la logística y el medio ambiente. Entre Ciencia e Ingeniería, **11**(22), 51–59 (2017). https://www.scielo.org.co/scielo.php?script=sci_arttext&pid=S1909-83672017000200051&lng=en&tlng=es. Accessed 03 Nov 2020
4. Orjuela-Castro, J.A., Suárez-Camelo, N., Chinchilla-Ospina, Y.I.: Costos logísticos y metodologías para el costeo en cadenas de suministro: una revisión de la literatura. Cuadernos de Contabilidad, **17**(44), 377–420 (2016). https://doi.org/10.11144/Javeriana.cc17-44.clmc
5. Johnson, M.P., Midgley, G., Chichirau, G.: Emerging trends and new frontiers in community operational research. Eur. J. Oper. Res. **268**(3), 1178–1191 (2018). https://doi.org/10.1016/j.ejor.2017.11.032
6. Mera, C.: UNAD Retos y Desafíos de la Prospectiva en las Organizaciones del Futuro, Grupo de Investigación y Estudios Prospectivos y Estrategicos (2019). ISBN 978–958–651–600–6
7. Dornier, P.-P., Ernst, R., Fender, M., Kouvelis, P.: Global Operations and Logistics: Text and Cases, Hardcover – January 1 1714 (1998)
8. Jordi Pau i Cos, Ricardo de Navascués y Gasca, Manual de logística integral, Madrid: EdicionesDíaz de Santos (2001). ISBN 84-7978-345-1
9. Roux, M.: Manual de logística para la gestión de almacenes. Gestión 2000, Barcelona (2003). ISBN 10: 8480881720

10. Ballou, R.: Logística administración de la cadena de suministro. Pearson Educación, México (2004). ISBN 970-26-0540-7
11. Carranza, O., Sabria, F.: Logística: mejores prácticas en Latinoamérica. Internacional Thomson Editores, México (2005). ISBN 13: 9789706864116
12. Christopher, M.: Logística aspectos estratégicos. Limusa, México (1999). ISBN 9789681852825
13. Casas, G.G., Romero, B.P.: Logística y distribución física: Evolución, situación actual, análisis comparativo y tendencias. Mc Graw-Hill.Interamericana, Madrid (1998). ISBN 84-481-1366-7
14. Smykay, E.W.: Physical Distribution Management: Logistics Problems of the Firm. Macmillan, New York (1961). A Macmillan marketing book (OCoLC) 614422824
15. Duran, S.: Liderazgo transformacional como estrategia de adaptación en la gestión logística empresarial. Revista Desarrollo Gerencial **4** (2017). https://doi.org/10.17081/dege.9.2
16. Farris, M.T.: Evolution of academic concerns with transportation and logistic. Transp. J. **37**, 42–50 (2017). https://www.jstor.org/stable/20713336
17. Chen, R., Liu, L., Wu, J.: Logistics capability and its grey assessment model. In: International Conference on IEEE Grey Systems and Intelligent Services (2007). https://doi.org/10.1109/GSIS.2007.4443455
18. Sanchez, O.: Guía para la construcción y análisis de indicadores, Departamento Nacional de Planeación, Bogota (2018)
19. BotthofErnst, A., Hartmann, A.: Zukunft der Arbeit im Kontext von Autonomik und Industrie 4.0. Zukunft der Arbeit in Industrie 4.0. Springer (2015). https://doi.org/10.1007/978-3-662-45915-7
20. BID: Logística Urbana: Los desafíos de la Distribución Urbana de Mercancías,» Centro de Estudios Económicos para el Desarrollo y la Competitividad , Cámara de comercio de Cartagena (2009). https://publications.iadb.org/es/publicacion/14260/logistica-urbana-los-desafios-de-la-distribucion-urbana-de-mercancias
21. de Lima, P., Orlem, B.S., Sandro, R.T., Manuel, C., Follmann, N.: Una nueva definición de la logística interna y forma de evaluar la misma. Ingeniare. Revista chilena de ingeniería **25**(2), 264–276 (2017). https://doi.org/10.4067/S0718-33052017000200264
22. La Rosa, V.: Resumén ejecutivo 2016 – 2019. Gobernación, Atlantico (2019)
23. Pérez: Sistemas de integración vertical y horizontal en el marco de industria 4.0: Evaluación y desarrollo. UANL, Monterrey (2017). https://eprints.uanl.mx/id/eprint/16246
24. Jung, K.: Mapping strategic goals and operational performance metrics for smart manufacturing systems. Procedia Comput. Sci. **44**, 184–193 (2015). https://doi.org/10.1016/j.procs.2015.03.051
25. Rennung, C.: Service Provision in the Framework of Industry 4.0. Procedia Soc. Behav. Sci. **221**, 372–377 (2016). https://doi.org/10.1016/j.sbspro.2016.05.127
26. Hernandez Sampieri, F.: Metodología de la Investigación. Mc Graw Hill, México (2014). ISBN 978-607-15-0291-9
27. Mejía, L.: Documentos CONPES consejo nacional de política económica y social república de Colombia departamento nacional de planeación, Bógota (2018). https://colaboracion.dnp.gov.co/CDT/Conpes/Econ%C3%B3micos/3918.pdf

Health Systems: Strategies for the Delimitation of Vulnerable Areas and Identification of Failures of Medical Equipment

Hub Location Problem for Medical Care During Epidemic Outbreaks

Jose Antonio Marmolejo-Saucedo[1]([⊠]) [iD] and Jorge Rojas-Arce[2] [iD]

[1] Facultad de Ingenieria, Universidad Panamericana,
Augusto Rodin 498, 03920 Ciudad de Mexico, Mexico
jmarmolejo@up.edu.mx
[2] Facultad de Ingenieria, Departamento de Ingenieria en Sistemas Biomedicos,
Universidad Nacional Auonoma de Mexico, Mexico City, Mexico
jorge.rojas.arce@comunidad.unam.mx

Abstract. This paper presents a proposal for the Hub location for medical care during epidemic outbreaks. A problem of coverage of medical services that offers a radius of medical attention to the population is analyzed. Two criteria are shown for the location of health services. Finally, based on public health policy recommendations, the solution is proposed for a hypothetical case.

Keywords: Facility location · Health systems · Supply chain

1 Literature Review

In the case of a Health system such as that of Mexico that has structural problems and a 70% full supply of medicines, facing a public health challenge such as the COVID-19 pandemic implies making value-added proposals that allow face contingencies like the current one. The design of a resilient medicine supply chain that can serve as a response to unexpected risks in the health system requires the participation of the different agents involved in the supply chain, in addition to the stewardship of the health department that allows the integration of wills and joint actions.

In the framework of an epidemic, it is necessary to guarantee medical supplies (medicines, vaccines, supplies, etc.) in addition to basic products (food, water, etc.). To guarantee the supply and supply of these products, it is necessary to have strategic storage and distribution centers that communicate with the expected demand points in the event of a contingency. It is precisely a problem of designing an emerging logistics network in the face of disruptive events. For this, it is necessary to define the number and location of distribution and collection centers, unloading places and the location of demand centers, and the selection of optimal distribution algorithms that guarantee the best performance of the network. As well as the definition of the required optimal inventory levels, replacement policies, transportation, and distribution according to the health contingency that is being faced.

© ICST Institute for Computer Sciences, Social Informatics and Telecommunications Engineering 2021
Published by Springer Nature Switzerland AG 2021. All Rights Reserved
J. A. Marmolejo-Saucedo et al. (Eds.): COMPSE 2020, LNICST 359, pp. 117–129, 2021.
https://doi.org/10.1007/978-3-030-69839-3_8

For the proper design of a network of this nature, it is necessary to have precise estimates of the demand required according to the contingency. Studies have been carried out combining demand estimation models related to epidemiological models of disease progression. Authors such as [5] propose a multi-objective programming model for the selection of emergency centers and the quantities of drugs to be transported from the supply sources to the demand points. In [14], they extend the vision of multi-objective programming towards a stochastic model using genetic algorithms for its solution. In [6], they integrate the analysis of system dynamics to model the dynamic behavior of the refueling, reception, and dispensing sources in the case of an anthrax attack. In [9], they propose a dynamic optimization model with variable replacement and transport times using heuristic methods for its solution. Other approaches consider logistics network designs with one-time supply and replenishment points [17]. Similarly, there are different versions of the modeling depending on the objective of the network, which can be to minimize inventory and transport costs or to minimize response time as a priority [15] and [19].

Various studies use the hybrid approach where they combine disease modeling through simulation and supply chain design through optimization models, [7] applies this approach to an anti-bioterrorism system. In [18], they analyze the distribution of medical supplies in affected areas considering a desirable minimum level of supply as well as maximum response times in addition to the associated costs. Similarly, vehicle routing problems are integrated into a context of epidemic control, works such as [4,8] and [12] have addressed this problem in their logistics designs.

In [2], they show the development of a coordinated supply chain for the distribution of the influenza vaccine. Taking into account the non-linear demand given the behavior of the disease and the most effective immunization strategies, combining the epidemiological model with the supply chain. In addition to the necessary coordination between the government and the vaccine provider, through shared risk schemes.

The study shows in [13] presents a systematic review of the health and disaster supply chain literature, especially in the case of natural disasters. They highlight the development of methodologies to abort the problem, based on operational management, information technology, inventory and control management, strategic management, and service management. As well as the application of new technologies for inventory management such as the use of RFID.

In [1], they develop a systematic review of relief distribution networks. Highlighting the contributions made about three stages defined in an emergency: a) preparedness and mitigation, b) response, and c) recovery. To attend to each stage, methodological contributions focused on location and network design, transportation (relief distribution and casualty transportation), and location and transportation are distinguished. Through exact and heuristic methods.

In [3], they present a literature review focused on epidemic control and logistics operations. Highlighting as a necessary attribute in the face of a health contingency the need for a quick response and coordination between the sectors involved to guarantee the supply of medical supplies, human and financial resources. Highlighting the time horizon in which you intervene, pre-event, or post-event. Bioterrorism, natural outbreaks, and disaster aftermath are considered as possible catastrophic events. The intervention considers as basic stages: 1) Preparedness, 2) Outbreak, 3) investigation, 4) Response, and 5) Evaluation. Table 1 shows the main logistical operations and decisions during the phases of an epidemic outbreak. The main methods used to analyze the problems associated with the health supply chain are simulation, game theory, mathematical modeling, economic analysis, cost-effectiveness analysis, optimization, and analysis of multi-criteria decisions.

Table 1. Most important logistics operations and decisions during the phases of the outbreak

Phase	Most important logistic operations
Preparedness	Identification of sources Contract management Inventory management Periodical review and updating of medical supplies Facility location of stockpiling centers Network design transportation/distribution Selection of facilities/health Availability of funds
Outbreak investigation	Provision of appropriate materials Training of clinical workers Provision of commodities and resources to the outbreak response Collection, transportation, and storage of specimens Procurement, handling, storing and distribution of laboratory commodities
Response	Selection of facilities (PODs) Review and updating of supplies Transportation/distribution of supplies and commodities Procurement of supplies once depleted Dispensing of medical supplies, supplementary materials, and commodities to the public Establishment of a cold supply chain for essential medical supplies Management of human resources Scheduling available vehicles Adjustments to the capacity of health care facilities to hospitalize infected people Management of patients in triage centers
Evaluation	Identification and assessments of possible bottlenecks of delays Evaluation of timelines that should have been respected Follow-up and monitoring of patients for the effectiveness of treatments Identification of patients requiring dose modification of alternative treatment Development of indicators to evaluate the performance of logistics control operations Assessment coordination issues Establishment and operation of rehabilitation procedures

A recent study by [16] analyzes a reverse logistics network design for the treatment of medical waste, in the framework of the COVID-19 pandemic in Wuhan (China). The study is of great importance due to the identification of a high rate of contagion as well as the residence time of the virus in objects that had contact with infected patients. Rapid response to the management of these wastes represents an opportunity to contain the spread of the epidemic. A multi-objective and multi-period model of mixed-integer programming is proposed for the design of the reverse logistics network.

The challenge is not less considering the complexity in the prediction of epidemic outbreaks, however, based on historical data, it has been possible to adequately model the probability of occurrence and possible scenarios of the magnitude of the problem. Stochastic variables and different simulation approaches must necessarily be included to obtain robust models. From a technical point of view, it is necessary to integrate innovative elements in supply chain management, such as the integration of:

- Multi-paradigm simulation schemes
- Discreet simulation
- Dynamic simulation
- Agent-based simulation
- Optimization algorithms
- Disruption event modeling
- Risk analysis in the supply chain

The use of data science tools, simulation, and optimization methodologies will allow efficient and timely management of the supply chain for medicines and supplies in a contingency. Currently, there is a specialized software that allows integrating different paradigms into hybrid models that allow generating technical evidence for public health decision-making.

2   Resilient Supply Chain Model

In this section, we develop the supply chain design model for a resilient supply network. We consider the model into a generalized network. The model is a mixed-integer linear problem.

Let K be the set of manufacturing plants. An element $k \in K$ identifies a specific plant of the company. Let I be the set of the potential cross-docking warehouses. An element $i \in I$ is a specific cross-docking warehouse. Finally, let J be the set of distribution centers, a specific distribution center is any $j \in J$. Let $\mathbb{Z}$ denote the set of integers $\{0,1\}$.

2.1   Parameters

Q_k = Capacity of plant k.
β_i = Capacity of cross-docking warehouse i.
F_i = Fixed cost of opening cross-docking warehouse in location i.
G_{ki} = Transportation cost per unit of the product from the plant k to the cross-docking warehouse i.
C_{ij} = Cost of shipping the product from the cross-dock i to the distribution center (CeDis) j.
d_j = Demand of the distribution center j.

2.2   Decision Variables

We have the following sets of binary variables to make the decisions about the opening of the cross-docking warehouse, and the distribution for the cross-docking warehouse to the distribution center.

$$Y_i = \begin{cases} 1 & \text{If location } i \text{ is used as a cross-docking warehouse,} \\ 0 & \text{otherwise,} \end{cases}$$

$$X_{ij} = \begin{cases} 1 & \text{If cross-dock } i \text{ supplies the demand of CeDis } j, \\ 0 & \text{otherwise,} \end{cases}$$

$W_{ki} = $ The amount of product sent from plant k to the cross-dock i is represented by continuous variables

We can now state the mathematical model as a (P) problem. See [10].

$$\min_{W_{ki}, Y_i, X_{ij}} Z = \sum_{k \in K} \sum_{i \in I} G_{ki} W_{ki} + \sum_{i \in I} F_i Y_i + \sum_{i \in I} \sum_{j \in J} C_{ij} d_j X_{ij} \tag{1}$$

Subject to constraints:

Capacity of the plant

$$\sum_{i \in I} W_{ki} \leq Q_k, \quad \forall k \in K \tag{2}$$

Balance of product

$$\sum_{j \in J} d_j X_{ij} = \sum_{k \in K} W_{ki}, \quad \forall i \in I \tag{3}$$

Single Cross-docking warehouse to distribution center

$$\sum_{i \in I} X_{ij} = 1, \quad \forall j \in J \tag{4}$$

Cross-docking warehouse capacity

$$\sum_{j \in J} d_j X_{ij} \leq \beta_i Y_i, \quad \forall i \in I \tag{5}$$

Demand of items

$$p Y_i \leq \sum_{k \in K} W_{ki}, \quad \forall i \in I \tag{6}$$

$$p = min\{d_j\} \tag{7}$$

$$W_{ki} \geq 0, \quad \forall i \in I, \forall k \in K \tag{8}$$

$$Y_i \in \mathbb{Z}, \quad \forall i \in I \tag{9}$$

$$X_{ij} \in \mathbb{Z}, \quad \forall i \in I, \forall j \in J \tag{10}$$

The objective function (1) considers in the first term the cost of shipping the product from the plant k to the cross-docking warehouse i. The second term contains the fix cost to open and operate the cross-docking warehouse i. The last term incorporates the cost of fulfilling the demand of the distribution center j. Constraint (2) implies that the output of plant k does not violate the capacity of plant k. Balance constraint (3) ensures that the amount of products that arrive to a distribution center j is the same as the products sent from the plant k. The demand of each distribution center j will be satisfied by a single cross-docking warehouse i, this is achieved by constraint (4). Constraint (5) bounds the amount of products that can be sent to a distribution center j from an opened cross-docking warehouse i. Constraint (6) guarantees that any opened cross-docking warehouse i receives at least the minimum amount of demand requested by a given distribution center j. Constraint (7) ensures that the minimum demand of each distribution center j is considered. Finally, constraints (8), (9) and (10) are the non-negative and integrality conditions.

3   Case Study

In this section, we describe the case study. In particular, we consider the pharmaceutical supply chain in Mexico. The supply chain is made up of four echelons: two factories, one central-distribution center, three regional-distribution centers and thirty-two wholesale drug distributors. These facilities and clients are scattered throughout the country. Figs. 1 and 2 represent the current structure of the supply chain.

The case study consists of finding a resilient solution that allows the supply chain to react efficiently to a disruption. The distribution centers will be the facilities subjected to hypothetical scenarios of disruption.

Table 2 shows the disruption scenarios considered.

All network diagrams were implemented in cytoscape software, see [11].

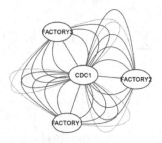

Fig. 1. CDC-Factory links.

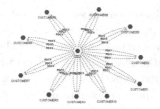

Fig. 2. CDC-RDC-CUSTOMER.

Table 2. Scenarios addressed in the case study

Scenario	Disruption	Breakdown time
I	One factory is closed due to health contingency	45 days
II	One DC is closed	30 days
III	All facilities are closed	15 days

3.1 Solution Methodology

The solution methodology used in this research is based on simulation-optimization. The anylogistix software was used to develop the "what if" methodology. This software uses CPLEX as an optimization engine to find the best solutions within a set of possible solutions. First, the current situation of the pharmaceutical company's supply chain is modeled. Subsequently, the elements or facilities that make up the supply network are optimized. Several operating policies of the chosen supply network are simulated. Finally, disruptive events are generated to test the resilience of the proposals to the previously defined disruption scenarios, see Fig. 3.

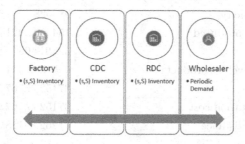

Fig. 3. Inventory policies and demand

3.2 Computational Results

Considering the three different scenarios, it was found that scenarios I and II are those that cause the greatest negative impact on the operation of the supply chain. For this, and for reasons of extension of the document, analysis of results shows the performance indicators for scenario I and scenario II. After running the optimization and simulation routines, the results obtained are as follows.

In the first instance, performance indicators for the current structure of the company were analyzed without disruption. Afterwards, the various scenarios were simulated. The variation experiment function, incorporated in ALX, was used to compare various key performance indicators. Figure 5 shows the current supply chain network structure.

For scenario I, the service level by product, the available inventory of all the facilities and the average delivery time are shown in Figs. 7, 8 and 9, respectively.

Scenario II, see Fig. 2, as mentioned above, was the one with the greatest disruptive effects and it is the scenario that generates less profits. As seen in Fig. 10, the level of service deteriorated to levels of 60% and 40% for each product. Figures 11 and 12, shows the available inventory and lead-time.

Once scenario II has been optimized, see Fig. 4, the results of the key performance indicators are reflected in Table 3. In this scenario, the highest profits are generated with a service level above 95%, see Fig. 13. The available inventory and lead time are shown in Figs. 14 and 15. Finally, the proposal to optimize scenario II is shown in Fig. 6.

Table 3. Key performance indicators of proposal solution

Available inventory	682342.6764	pcs
Demand (Products backlog)	0	pcs
Demand placed (Products) by customer	1061896.722	pcs
Demand received (Products)	2483056.467	pcs
Fulfillment received (Products On-time)	1050395.745	pcs
Fulfillment received (Products)	1421159.745	pcs
Fulfillment shipped (Orders)	393	Order
Peak capacity	989528	pcs
Products produced	1545502.421	pcs
Profit	3.52E+08	USD
Service level by products	0.989169401	Ratio
Total cost	3715253.767	USD
Transportation cost	3715253.767	USD
Traveled distance	41252.88728	km

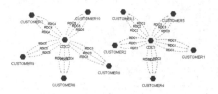

Fig. 4. Several CDCs.

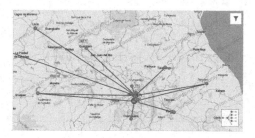

Fig. 5. Current supply chain network.

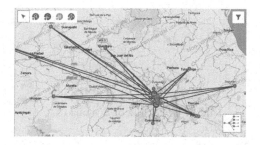

Fig. 6. Supply chain network proposal.

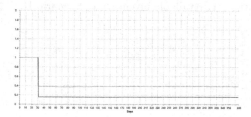

Fig. 7. Service level of Scenario I.

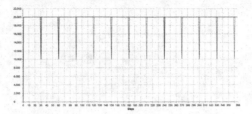

Fig. 8. Available inventory of Scenario I.

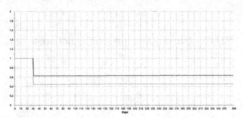

Fig. 9. Lead-time of Scenario I.

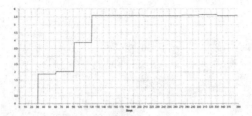

Fig. 10. Service level of Scenario II.

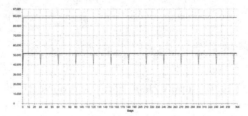

Fig. 11. Available inventory of Scenario II.

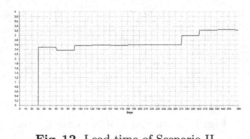

Fig. 12. Lead-time of Scenario II.

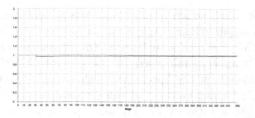

Fig. 13. Service level of Scenario II optimized.

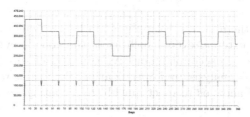

Fig. 14. Available inventory of Scenario II optimized.

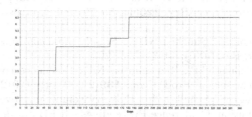

Fig. 15. Lead-time of Scenario II optimized.

4   Conclusions

According to the scenarios outlined for the company, the epidemic outbreak of COVID-19 in Mexico caused several disruptions in the supply chain of medicines.

The solution methodology based on a simulation-optimization approach, allows analyzing the impacts of the different recovery strategies for a subsequent epidemiological outbreak. Additionally, the proposed approach allows enable a comprehensive view of the supply network, as well as fast and efficient responses to risky situations and changing.

Mexico has great health challenges, it is going through a demographic and epidemiological transition where chronic degenerative diseases predominate. The public sector medicine supply chain in Mexico has several structural problems related to the characteristics of the Health System. In 2018, the percentage of a full supply of medications represented 70%, historically maintaining a percentage of prescriptions not filled, which implies that the patient must expend out-of-pocket expenses to acquire their medications or not take treatment.

Starting from this deficient structure of the medicine supply chain in the public sector, facing an epidemic such as the case of COVID-19 represents a very important challenge for the Mexican health system. The present pandemic has represented a significant increase in the demand for public health services. As of April 28, 2020, a total of 77 thousand probable cases were registered in the epidemiological surveillance system, of which 16,752 cases were positive with COVID-19. The crude mortality rate represented 93.3 deaths per 1000 inhabitants, and adults and older adults with some chronic disease are mainly affected.

In this context, the need for a supply chain for medicines and supplies that allows dealing with external events such as a pandemic is evident. For this, it is necessary to take into account innovative concepts of supply chain management, simulation, risk analysis, and optimization. Being able to have robust and efficient designs will allow us to react quickly to a contingency.

References

1. Anaya-Arenas, A.M., Renaud, J., Ruiz, A.: Relief distribution networks: a systematic review. Ann. Oper. Res. **223**(1), 53–79 (2014). https://doi.org/10.1007/s10479-014-1581-y
2. Chick, S.E., Mamani, H., Simchi-Levi, D.: Supply chain coordination and influenza vaccination. Oper. Res. **56**(6), 1493–1506 (2008)
3. Dasaklis, T.K., Pappis, C.P., Rachaniotis, N.P.: Epidemics control and logistics operations: a review. Int. J. Prod. Econ. **139**(2), 393–410 (2012)
4. Herrmann, J., Riggs, S., Schalliol, K.: Delivery volume improvement for planning medication distribution. Conference Proceedings - IEEE International Conference on Systems, Man and Cybernetics, pp. 3505–3509, October 2009. https://doi.org/10.1109/ICSMC.2009.5346773
5. Hu, J., Zhao, L.: Emergency logistics network based on integrated supply chain response to public health emergency. ICIC Express Lett. **6**, 113–118 (2012)
6. Hu, J., Zhao, L.: Emergency logistics strategy in response to anthrax attacks based on system dynamics. Int. J. Math. Oper. Res. **3**, 490–509 (2011). https://doi.org/10.1504/IJMOR.2011.042440
7. Ke, Y., Zhao, L.: Optimization of emergency logistics delivery model based on anti-bioterrorism. In: 2008 IEEE International Conference on Industrial Engineering and Engineering Management, pp. 2077–2081. IEEE (2008)
8. Liu, M., Zhao, L.: Optimization of the emergency materials distribution network with time windows in anti-bioterrorism system. Int. J. Innov. Comput. Inf. Control **5**, 3615–3624 (2009)
9. Liu, M., Zhao, L.: An integrated and dynamic optimisation model for the multi-level emergency logistics network in anti-bioterrorism system. Int. J. Syst. Sci. **43**, 1464–1478 (2012). https://doi.org/10.1080/00207721.2010.547629
10. Marmolejo, J., Rodríguez, R., Cruz-Mejia, O., Saucedo, J.: Design of a distribution network using primal-dual decomposition. Math. Probl. Eng. **2016**, 9 (2016)
11. Shannon, P., et al.: Cytoscape: a software environment for integrated models of biomolecular interaction networks. Genome Res. **13**(11), 2498–2504 (2003)

12. Shen, Z., Dessouky, M., Ordóñez, F.: A two-stage vehicle routing model for large-scale bioterrorism emergencies. Networks **54**, 255–269 (2009). https://doi.org/10.1002/net.20337
13. Syahrir, I., Suparno, S., Vanany, I.: Healthcare and disaster supply chain: literature review and future research. Proc. Manuf. **4**, 2–9 (2015). https://doi.org/10.1016/j.promfg.2015.11.007
14. Wang, H., Wang, X., Zeng, A.: Optimal material distribution decisions based on epidemic diffusion rule and stochastic latent period for emergency rescue. International Journal of Mathematics in Operational Research 1 (2009). https://doi.org/10.1504/IJMOR.2009.022876
15. Xu, J., Zhao, L., Wang, H.: Collaborative research between epidemic diffusion network and emergency rescue network in anti-bioterrorism system. In: 2009 International Joint Conference on Computational Sciences and Optimization, vol. 2, pp. 630–634. IEEE (2009)
16. Yu, H., Sun, X., Solvang, W.D., Zhao, X.: Reverse logistics network design for effective management of medical waste in epidemic outbreaks: Insights from the coronavirus disease 2019 (covid-19) outbreak in wuhan (china). Int. J. Environ. Res. Public Health **17**(5), 1770 (2020). https://doi.org/10.3390/ijerph17051770
17. Zhao, L., Sun, L.: Emergency service modes of supply chains with replenishment sources. In: 2008 International Conference on Service Systems and Service Management, pp. 1–7 (2008)
18. Zhao, W., Han, R.: Optimal model of emergency relief supplies distribution in anti-bioterrorism system. In: 2010 International Conference on Logistics Systems and Intelligent Management, ICLSIM 2010, vol. 3, January 2010. https://doi.org/10.1109/ICLSIM.2010.5461244
19. Zhu, L., Cao, J.: A network equilibrium model for emergency logistics response under disaster spreading. In: 2010 International Conference on Logistics Engineering and Intelligent Transportation Systems, LEITS2010 - Proceedings, November 2010. https://doi.org/10.1109/LEITS.2010.5664931

Application of Spectral Clustering
for the Detection of High Priority Areas
of Attention for COVID-19 in Mexico

Rodriguez-Aguilar Roman(✉) (iD)

Facultad de Ciencias Económicas y Empresariales, Universidad Panamericana,
Augusto Rodin 498, 03920 Mexico City, Mexico
rrodrigueza@up.edu.mx

Abstract. The recent COVID-19 pandemic has represented a great challenge for
health systems around the world. That is why it is necessary to propose strategies
for prioritizing care and containing the pandemic. This work proposes the use
of spectral clustering to characterize high-priority areas of care based on key
information on the performance of the pandemic as well as health system variables.
The result shows the generation of high priority areas not only due to the deaths
observed but also due to the clinical, demographic and health system variables.

Keywords: Unsupervised models · Spectral cluster · COVID-19 · Priorization ·
Mexico

1 Introduction

The COVID-19 pandemic that we are currently experiencing has generated multiple
effects at the health and economic level. In most countries, contingency plans were
developed in the health systems to meet the growing demand for health services for
pandemic care. The need for more resources in the health sector is evident and therefore
also requires strategic planning of the allocation of these resources. The challenges have
arisen in various dimensions, from being able to guarantee access to inputs and human
resources to defining strategies to contain the wave of infections. At a technical level in
various countries, various studies have emerged that allow evaluating both the impact
and possible strategies for solving the contingencies observed in health systems. An
essential point in these studies is the prioritization of the susceptible population and
the infected population at the regional level in the countries. It is important to focus
resources on those priority areas that make it possible to avoid an increase in infections
as well as guarantee access to medical care for patients who require second and third
level care.

The research carried out during the pandemic are grouped into strategies for the
containment of the pandemic. The World Health Organization issued in June 2020
the document entitled "Maintaining essential health services: operational guidance for
the COVID-19 context", where it addresses strategic aspects and recommendations for

J. A. Marmolejo-Saucedo et al. (Eds.): COMPSE 2020, LNICST 359, pp. 130–142, 2021.
https://doi.org/10.1007/978-3-030-69839-3_9

nations to overcome the current health crisis, among the main aspects The maintenance of the essential operations of the health services is highlighted, through the coordination of the different actors, as well as the prioritization of essential services that allow adaptation to each context and needs. Guaranteeing essential drugs, equipment and supplies is a fundamental element, as well as establishing emerging financing mechanisms that guarantee the availability of resources. Strengthen monitoring, communication as well as the use of digital platforms to support essential health service delivery [1]. [2] proposes a strategy for the containment of the pandemic based on four main axes, stopping the international and national flow of passengers, creating administrative zones per million people, stopping unnecessary flow between non-emergency zones except for the transport of goods, as well as establishing an information-driven value chain of services to control the spread of the pandemic within an area. [3] analyze demand scenarios for hospital beds, as well as assisted ventilation equipment, according to different scenarios for the Brazilian health system. The results show a saturation of the Brazilian health system, due to the fact that various health microregions and macro regions would operate beyond their capacity. The construction of field hospitals is important, both in places where there are historically healthcare gaps, as well as in those where there is already pressure from demand. The third message refers to the regional organization of health services that, despite being adequate in situations of habitual demand, in times of pandemic, this design implies additional challenges, especially if the distance that the patient had to travel was very far. To inform Canada's response to COVID-19, a rapid-cycle priority identification process was conducted. Seven COVID-19 priorities were identified for health services and policy research: adaptation of the system and organization of care; decision making and ethics on resource allocation; rapid synthesis and comparative policy analysis of COVID-19 response and outcomes; sanitary workforce; virtual care; long-term consequences of the pandemic; and public and patient participation. Three additional cross-cutting themes were identified: supporting the health of indigenous peoples and vulnerable populations, digital and data infrastructure, and learning from health systems and knowledge platforms [4].

Clinical studies focused on the analysis of the pandemic as well as possible treatments and the subsequent development of a vaccine. [5] analyze the main clinical treatments used so far to treat the disease through a systematic literature review. [6] raises the need to establish a set of public health interventions to mitigate the spread of the epidemic, taking the Italian case as a reference, establishing possible scenarios of the pandemic for Canada. On the other hand, issues related to the economic and social impacts due to the pandemic are addressed, a part of these studies focus on the analysis of supply chains for supplies and medicines, as well as different sectors economically affected by the pandemic. [7] Analyze at drug supply networks facing shortage challenges in many situations, such as current outbreaks like COVID-19. Drug shortages can occur due to manufacturing problems, lack of infrastructure, and immediate reaction mechanisms. A hypothetical case study is presented using optimization and simulation algorithms to observe the impact of COVID-19 on a regional supply network. [8] evaluates the main implications of COVID-19 on drug shortages, emphasizing the need for international and regional collaboration, as well as communication and flexibility within health systems. The risks that the current pandemic represents for timely access to medicines not only related to the pandemic are of great relevance for the correct management of the pandemic as well as for the correct management of future health crises. [9] addresses the potential benefits of using artificial intelligence and internet of things methods to prevent the spread of COVID-19 through a systematic review of the main applications and scope that artificial intelligence could have in the prevention and control of the pandemic. [10] propose the planning and operation of alternative care centers in disaster response situations should include the participation of pharmacists in key decision-making processes in the early planning stages. [11] show the potential application of simulation models to reduce the impact of COVID-19, highlighting the management of resources within specific regions, considering in an integral way the clinical care process as well as the timely access to the necessary resources to face the pandemic.

In the case of Mexico, there is a fragmented health system, linked to the patient's employment situation. There are three major public health systems: the IMSS (Mexican Institute of Social Security) linked to the population that works in the private sector, the ISSSTE (Institute of Social Security and Services of State Workers, for its acronym in Spanish) and INSABI (Institute of Health for Wellbeing, for its acronym in Spanish) that serves the rest of the open population and that replaced the Seguro Popular. In addition to having a fragmented health system, Mexico has an extensive and dispersed territory, which complicates logistics operations to guarantee timely access to medicines and supplies in a health context like the current one. The Mexican territory is characterized by its diversity and population dispersion, there are remote communities in the mountains of difficult access. Historically, health strategies have been defined to be able to access these remote communities, but in the framework of the COVID-19 pandemic, these operations are seen as an important challenge for the Mexican health system, which is why a prioritization mechanism is proposed region of high priority areas for pandemic care.

The health ministry has defined health jurisdictions that allow it to plan resources as well as access to health services. The Sanitary Jurisdiction is a regional administrative unit constituted based on demographic, epidemiological, geographical, political and social criteria. It brings together rural and urban municipalities and has health centers, specialized medical units, hospitals and other organizations to develop prevention and health protection programs and services. In the context of the current pandemic, it is necessary to structure the organization and allocation of resources based on the characteristics of each region affected by the pandemic, which requires the use of care areas that may not be organized within the framework of a jurisdiction sanitary. However, it is necessary to define these priority areas, albeit temporarily, in order to focus efforts and resources to contain the pandemic and guarantee access to medical care in a timely manner for the affected population, as well as establish strategies to contain the pandemic. The objective of this research is to propose the use of an unsupervised machine learning model for the prioritization of areas of attention for COVID-19, considering fundamental elements such as the availability of human resources and infrastructure, as well as the behavior of the pandemic throughout the Mexican territory. The work is structured as follows, in the first section the status of the pandemic in Mexico is addressed using statistics issued by the Ministry of Health, about tests carried out, number of infections and deaths, as well as mortality rates by groups old. The next section addresses the methodology to be used and the main sources of information. Finally, the results are presented as well as the main conclusions and recommendations of the study.

2   COVID-19 Pandemic in Mexico

The impact of the pandemic in Mexico has been differentiated according to the health conditions of the patients as well as regional aspects. The information available as of October 2020 published by the Ministry of Health shows a total of one million possible cases, of which 52% were confirmed as positive. The proportion of men with respect to women has a higher incidence, in the same way two categories are integrated in addition to positive and non-positive cases, which are inappropriate results (referring to problems with the tests) as well as cases outside the sample (Fig. 1). The increase in the number of cases and deaths has been consistent since the beginning of the pandemic, in recent months no evidence has been identified that indicates that the pandemic has happened in Mexico.

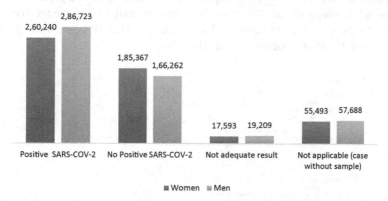

Fig. 1. Total cases registered as of October 2020. Source: Ministry of Health of Mexico.

When analyzing the distribution by federal entity, a higher incidence of confirmed cases is observed in Mexico City, the State of Mexico, Guanajuato, Nuevo León and Veracruz as the states with the highest number of confirmed cases. These five states account for 44% of the total confirmed cases throughout the country. For their part, the states with the lowest number of cases are Colima, Nayarit, Morelos, Zacatecas and Campeche with only 4% of the total confirmed cases (Fig. 2).

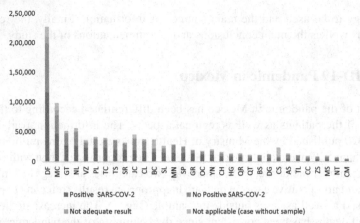

Fig. 2. Total cases registered as of October 2020 by state. Source: Ministry of Health of Mexico.

The distribution of cases by age group shows a concentration of a greater number of cases in people between 25 and 54 years of age, concentrating 63% of the total confirmed cases. The lowest incidence of cases is observed in ages 0 to 19 years with less with a participation of 4% of all confirmed cases (Fig. 3).

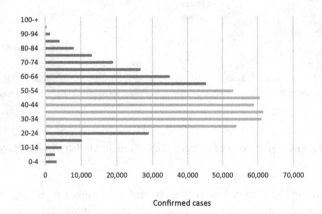

Confirmed cases

Fig. 3. Total confirmed as of October 2020, cases per five-year age. Source: Ministry of Health of Mexico.

Mortality by age groups is more vulnerable to age groups over 60 years of age, with an average rate of 407 deaths per thousand inhabitants. The lowest mortality rates are found in young population groups aged 0 to 34 years with an average of 14 deaths per thousand inhabitants (Fig. 4). It is important to identify the populations at risk by age and based on this information to be able to focus efforts by the health system.

It is clear that the pandemic in Mexico has not reached its peak and is far from having been overcome. For this reason, it is important to analyze possible scenarios and action strategies using technically robust tools to be able to solve in the best possible way this great challenge for the Mexican health system. It is important to emphasize that

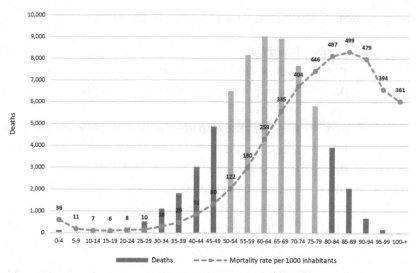

Fig. 4. Mortality rate per thousand inhabitants per five-year age. Source: Ministry of Health of Mexico.

the information used is the available information published by the Ministry of Health, which could be modified due to the constant registration and validation activities. In addition to the incidence of cases, it is important to take into account the severity of these and their demand for specialized health services, according to the information from the Ministry of Health of the total of confirmed patients as of October 2020, 74% correspond to outpatient cases and 26% to cases that required hospitalization. Of the total number of hospitalized patients, 9% required the use of intensive care units and 19% required to be intubated.

3   Materials and Methods

The objective of the work is to identify high priority areas of attention for the COVID-19 pandemic throughout the Mexican territory, it seeks to integrate information regarding the evolution of the pandemic as well as variables related to the state of the health system of each federative entity, taking into account the availability of infrastructure, human and financial resources, as well as epidemiological aspects of the populations served.

3.1   Description of the Data

The information used corresponds to the last available cut-off regarding resources and infrastructure, there is a lag in the availability of information on the health sector, so the latest information available on these items corresponds to the year 2019. Additionally, corresponding variables were integrated to the evolution of the pandemic, for which there are records from January to October 2020. Table 1 shows the variables considered according to each item of analysis, four essential items are considered: 1) health resources, 2) services provided, 3) health spending and 4) evolution of the pandemic.

Table 1. Variables considered in five dimensions of analysis.

Variable	Description
TPS	Total public spending on health
DN	Doctors and nurses in contact with the patient
MU	Medical units
BDS	Beds in the hospitalization area
ICU	Intensive care units
HD	Hospital discharges
NDD	Noncommunicable disease discharges
CPC	COVID-19 positive cases
CDTH	COVID-19 deaths

The information considered is key for estimating the groups to be served with higher priority according to their structural characteristics, in addition to the incidence and deaths of patients from COVID-19. The disaggregation of information is only available at the state level for all variables, it would be ideal to have more disaggregated information at the municipality level, but this proposal can be a reference for future studies that allow a higher level of disaggregation.

3.2 Spectral Cluster Analysis

The use of an unsupervised machine learning model is proposed, because there is no previous antecedent of a classification of this nature. The objective is to identify specific patterns according to the profiles of the states in relation to the severity of the pandemic in those states. Within the available cluster analysis methodologies, the spectral cluster was considered as a classification method given its methodological characteristics that allow the identification of a data structure that does not necessarily present groupings with no conventional boundaries. One of the advantages of the spectral cluster is that it uses a similarity measure which is less restrictive than a distance measure, this allows generating more flexible clusters.

The spectral grouping method uses the information from the data similarity matrix to perform the dimensionality reduction. Using the similarity matrix as input, each pair of points in the data set is evaluated. This methodology considers that the points to be grouped are not part of a space vector. The variables to consider or the attributes are incorporated in a single dimension, the similarity, which takes a numerical value for each pair of points (i, j). Given a set of data, the similarity matrix can be defined as a symmetric matrix A, where $A_{ij} \geq 0$ represents a measure of similarity between data points (i, j). The general approach for spectral clustering is to use a standard clustering method (usually K-means or K-medoids) on relevant eigenvectors of a Laplacian matrix of A. There are several ways to define a Laplacian with different mathematical interpretations, so spectral groupings will also have different interpretations. Relevant eigenvectors are those that correspond to several smaller Laplacian eigenvalues. The main goal of spectral clustering is to find the global clustering of the data set that emerges from the pairwise interactions of its points. Namely, we want to put points that are similar to each other in the same cluster, dissimilar points in different clusters [12].

The concepts based on graph theory is generally used for the spectral cluster. Let the points to be grouped be $V = (1, \ldots, n)$ nodes of a graph G, and the graph edges be represented by the pairs (i, j) with $A_{ij} \geq 0$. Similarity is the weight of edge ij.

$$G = (V, E), E = \{(i,j), A_{ij} > 0\} \subseteq V \times V \tag{1}$$

G is an undirected and weighted graph. A partition of nodes of the graph in K participles or clusters was known as (K-way) graph cut. Therefore, the spectral clustering can be seen as the search for slices in the graph G. In addition to the similarity matrix, there is a set of derived matrices that are a fundamental part of the spectrum cluster methodology. One of the main matrices used is the Normalized Laplacian matrix, which is defined as follows.

$$L_{(n \times n)} = I - D^{-1/2} A D^{-1/2} \tag{2}$$

Where, A is a similarity matrix, $D = diag(d_1, \ldots, d_n)$ is a diagonal matrix for the node degrees and I is the unit matrix and $P = D^{-1}A$ is a random walk matrix. Based on the information captured by the similarity matrix and the Laplacian matrix, the objective of the spectral cluster is to project the information in a space of less dimension where the segmentation of the groups is natural and allows groups to be adjusted to unconventional forms. A generalized version of the spectral clustering algorithm is shown below [13, 14].

```
Algorithm Spectral Clustering
Input Similarity matrix A, number of clusters K
    1. Transform A
       Calculate di ← Σⁿⱼ₌₁ Aᵢⱼ, j =1: n the node degrees.
       From the transition matrix P with Pᵢⱼ ← Aᵢⱼ/dᵢ, for i,j =1: n
    2. Eigen-decomposition
       Compute the largest K eigenvalues λ₁ ≥ ⋯ ≥ λK and ei-
       genvectors V₁,... VK of P.
    3. Embed the data in K − th principal subspace
       Let xᵢ = [Vᵢ₂ Vᵢ₃ ... VᵢK] ∈ Rⁿˣ⁽K⁻¹⁾, for i =1,... n.
    4. Run the K-means algorithm of the data x₁:ₙ
       Output the clustering C obtained in step 4.
```

Among the main applications of the spectral cluster methodology are image recognition [15], image segmentation [16], urban land use [17], network community detection [18], speech separation [19], and demand response applications [20].

4 Results

4.1 Priorization of States for COVID-19 Attention

When estimating the similarity matrix and the Laplacian matrix of these, it is possible to extract the eigenvectors that represent the projection of the data in a smaller dimension, in this case it is observed that with the first two eigenvectors the greater amount of information of the dimension is represented original, it is decided to keep the first two dimensions of the spectral decomposition. Figure 5 shows the eigenvalues of each eigenvector of the Laplacian graph. In this case, the largest gap is between the eigenvectors 2 and 3, so a K = 4 would correspond. But nevertheless, in this case, three partitions were selected to be able to consider a pandemic monitoring semaphore in terms of selecting those states that represent the highest priority, entities on alert and entities without significant risks.

The first three dimensional eigenvectors of the spectral decomposition will be used to run the K-means algorithm with three partitions. With the information generated from the spectral cluster, three partitions were generated using a K-means algorithm, and the t-SNE 3D algorithm (t-Distributed Stochastic Neighbor Embedding) was applied to observe the separation in the projected space through spectral decomposition, we can observe that the three groups sought are clearly segmented in a three-dimensional space (Fig. 6).

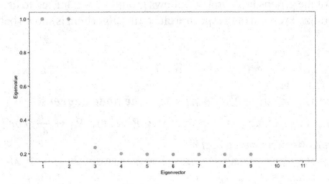

Fig. 5. Eigenvalues of each eigenvector of the Laplacian graph.

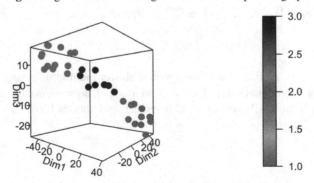

Fig. 6. t-SNE 3D graph for the three partitions.

Table 2. Profile of the clusters generated (average values for each variable)

Cluster	States	TPS*	DN	MU	BDS	ICU	HD	NDD	CPC	CDTH
I	AS, BS, CC, CM, DG, MS, NT, QT, QR, TL, ZS	7,117,448	6,466	298	912	5	69,879	27,985	5,336	5,356
II	BC, CS, CH, DF, GT, JC, MC, MN, NL, PL, SR, TS, VZ	34,386,594	28,307	981	4,849	23	288,100	134,068	28,428	28,744
III	CL, GR, HG, OC, SP, SL, TC, YN	14,060,391	13,413	810	2,062	11	143,021	57,138	14,838	14,869

* Thousands of pesos.

According to the three groups generated, it can be seen that they meet the objective, states with the highest incidence and mortality in COVID-19 are grouped, which present problems of resource availability as well as high values in associated diseases as a risk factor. Table 2 shows the profiles identified for each generated group, group I contains 11 states, group I is made up of 13 states, and group III contains 8 states. Group I corresponds to the states with lower risk, these are states with low health resources but also with low incidence and deaths from COVID-19, an interesting aspect of this group is the low incidence in discharges related to chronic diseases non-transmissible, in addition to being relatively small states in size and population, so the risk of contagion due to high population density is lower. Group II corresponds to the largest entities that in turn concentrate greater resources in health and greater risks related to chronic non-communicable diseases, in addition to presenting the highest incidence and deaths from

COVID-19, in this case a particular characteristic in Mexico is since the flow of patients is generally concentrated in the largest cities, the data corresponding to confirmed cases and deaths from COVID-19 correspond to the entity where the medical unit where the patient was treated is located and not to their state of origin. Group III corresponds to entities with lower risk with moderate health resources as well as confirmed patients and deaths from COVID-19.

It is important to note that the results generated are based on the information available on the pandemic so far, so they are subject to the quality of the information available. However, the methodological structure is applicable for detailed and reliable information that may not be public at the moment.

5 Conclusions

The pandemic that we are currently experiencing has generated the need to propose and implement innovative ideas for its management and attention to the problems related to the attention of COVID-19. Mexico is no exception since the rate of infections and deaths has been increasing since the first months. A fundamental element for the correct management and overcoming of this crisis is the efficient and timely allocation of health resources that allow to face this crisis.

Various studies have been developed worldwide in relation to the care of the health crisis, from different perspectives, most of them focused on the clinical care of the pandemic, but a significant proportion seeks to solve the problems directly and indirectly linked to the health crisis, such as streamlining logistics processes to ensure timely access to health resources, the development of simulation models and artificial intelligence that allow defining the most efficient and effective strategies to contain contagions as well as to avoid saturation of health services. It is precisely in this sense that the present work seeks to provide technical evidence for decision-making, integrating an unsupervised support model based on spectral clustering.

The application of a spectral clustering model makes it possible to address the grouping of states in the Mexican republic, allowing the integration of structures with unconventional borders, by projecting an n-dimensional space in a low-dimensional space through the use of the similarity matrix and the Laplace matrix. The results generated show congruence, three groups are identified based on the availability of health resources as well as the risk due to the growing demand for medical care and deaths from COVID-19, identifying the priority states will allow a more efficient and targeted allocation of resources to be able to act strategically in the face of the current contingency. In the same way, the results generated can serve as antecedent for a much more disaggregated grouping and with a greater number of variables that allow the allocation of resources to be focused even more. However, it is necessary to have detailed information in a timely manner to achieve this goal.

Annex

See Table 3.

Table 3. Catalog of federative entities of the Mexican Republic.

State	Abbreviation
AGUASCALIENTES	AS
BAJA CALIFORNIA	BC
BAJA CALIFORNIA SUR	BS
CAMPECHE	CC
COAHUILA DE ZARAGOZA	CL
COLIMA	CM
CHIAPAS	CS
CHIHUAHUA	CH
CIUDAD DE MÉXICO	DF
DURANGO	DG
GUANAJUATO	GT
GUERRERO	GR
HIDALGO	HG
JALISCO	JC
MÉXICO	MC
MICHOACÁN DE OCAMPO	MN
MORELOS	MS
NAYARIT	NT
NUEVO LEÓN	NL
OAXACA	OC
PUEBLA	PL
QUERÉTARO	QT
QUINTANA ROO	QR
SAN LUIS POTOSÍ	SP
SINALOA	SL
SONORA	SR
TABASCO	TC
TAMAULIPAS	TS
TLAXCALA	TL
VERACRUZ	VZ
YUCATÁN	YN
ZACATECAS	ZS

References

1. World Health Organization. (2020). Maintaining essential health services: operational guidance for the COVID-19 context: interim guidance, 1 June 2020. World Health Organization
2. Baveja, A., Kapoor, A., Melamed, B.: Stopping Covid-19: a pandemic-management service value chain approach. Ann. Oper. Res. **289**, 173–184 (2020)
3. Noronha, K.V, et al.: Pandemia por COVID-19 no Brasil: análise da demanda e da oferta de leitos hospitalares e equipamentos de ventilação assistida segundo diferentes cenários. Cadernos de Saúde Pública, **36**(6), e00115320. Epub 17 June 2020
4. McMahon, M., Nadigel, J., Thompson, E., Glazier, R.H.: Informing Canada's Health System Response to COVID-19: Priorities for Health Services and Policy Research. Healthcare policy = Politiques de sante, **17**(1), 112–124 (2020)
5. Hussain, S., Xie, Y., Li, D., et al.: Current strategies against COVID-19. Chin. Med. **15**, 70 (2020)
6. Scarabel, F., Pellis, L., Bragazzi, N.L., Wu, J.: Canada needs to rapidly escalate public health interventions for its COVID-19 mitigation strategies. Infect. Dis. Model. **5**, 316–322 (2020)
7. Lozano-Diez, J.A., MS, J.A., Rodriguez-Aguilar, R.: Designing a resilient supply chain: an approach to reduce drug shortages in epidemic outbreaks. PHAT, EAI (2020)
8. Shuman, A.G., Fox, E., Unguru, Y.: Preparing for COVID-19-related drug shortages. Ann. Am. Thorac. Soc. **17**(8), 928–931 (2020)
9. Adly, A.S., Adly, A.S., Adly, M.S.: Approaches based on artificial intelligence and the internet of intelligent things to prevent the spread of COVID-19: scoping review. J. Med. Internet Res. **22**(8), e19104 (2020)
10. Nelsen, G., et al.: Considerations for development of pharmacy support models for COVID-19 alternate care sites. Am. J. Health-Syst. Pharm. **77**(19), 1592–1597 (2020)
11. Currie, C.S.M., et al.: How simulation modelling can help reduce the impact of COVID-19. J. Simul. **14**(2), 83–97 (2020)
12. Meila, M.: Spectral Clustering: A Tutorial for the 2010's, pp. 1–23. CRC Press, Boca Raton (2016)
13. Meila, M., Shi, J.: Learning segmentation by random walks. Adv. Neural. Inf. Process. Syst. **13**, 873–879 (2001)
14. Meila, M., Shi, J.: A random walks view of spectral segmentation. In: Jaakkola, T., Richardson, T., (eds.), Artificial Intelligence and Statistics AISTATS (2001b)
15. Tolliver, D.A., Miller, G..: Graph partitioning by spectral rounding: applications in image segmentation and clustering. In: IEEE Computer Society Conference on Computer Vision and Pattern Recognition (CVPR 2006), New York, NY, USA, 2006, pp. 1053–1060 (2006)
16. Schultz, T., Kindlmann, G.L.: Open-box spectral clustering: applications to medical image analysis. IEEE Trans. Vis. Comput. Graph. **19**(12), 2100–2108 (2013)
17. Frias-Martinez, V., Frias-Martinez, E.: Spectral clustering for sensing urban land use using twitter activity. Eng. Appl. Artif. Intell. **35**, 237–245 (2014)
18. Shen, G., Ye, D.: A distance-based spectral clustering approach with applications to network community detection. J. Ind. Inf. Integr. **6**, 22–32 (2017)
19. Bach, F.R., Jordan, M.: Learning spectral clustering, with application to speech separation. J. Mach. Learn. Res. **7**(71), 1963–2001 (2006)
20. Lin, S., Li, F., Tian, E., Fu, Y., Li, D.: Clustering load profiles for demand response applications. IEEE Trans. Smart Grid **10**(2), 1599–1607 (2019)

Identifying the Main Causes of Medical Devices Failures While Surgery at High Specialization Hospital Implementing Lean Six Sigma

Ana Paula Yañez-Brand[1]([envelope]) [iD], Zaida E. Alarcón-Bernal[1] [iD], Javier Pérez-Orive[2] [iD],
and Eloy A. Hernández Lorenzo[2] [iD]

[1] Universidad Nacional Autónoma de México, Universidad 3000, 04510 Mexico City, Mexico
anapybrand@gmail.com, zaida.alarcon@unam.mx
[2] Instituto Nacional de Rehabilitación Luis Guillermo Ibarra Ibarra, Calz Mexio-Xochimilco 289, 14389 Mexico City, Mexico
jperezoribe.inr@gmail.com, eloyhl@yahoo.com.mx

Abstract. This project leads through the implementation of Lean Six Sigma (LSS) at two Surgical Units (SU) of the National Rehabilitation Institute (INR), a public high specialty Mexican hospital, to analyze and identify the main causes that produce failures in Medical Devices (MDs) during surgery. We applied the first three stages DMAIC methodology and LSS tools to achieve it. In the Define stage, the problematic was described. In the following stage, Measure, waste was identified on the work routine of the Biomedical Engineer (BE), who is part of the Biomedical Engineering Department (BED), with a Value Stream Map (VSM). In the final stage, Analyze, the causes of the principal ideas provided in the previous steps were determined. We identified the strongest factors that affect the processes involved in the elimination of mistakes or failures with MDs and waste. We studied these factors to understand their principal causes, to analyze them. Finally, we identified the main causes that produce MD failures during routine surgeries in the two SUs.

Keywords: Lean Six Sigma · Healthcare system · Quality improvement · Surgical unit · Biomedical engineering · Medical devices

1 Introduction

Mexican healthcare system is established by two sectors: public and private. The private sector provides services to the population with the ability to pay. The public sector includes social security institutions that provide services to workers, and institutions that protect or provide services to the population without social security [1]. The public sector has three levels of hospitals in health services.

The first level carries out actions to promote and protect the health, disease prevention, early diagnosis of damage, and outpatient care for the most frequent morbidity provided by general practitioners and nursing personnel. The second level provides basic

J. A. Marmolejo-Saucedo et al. (Eds.): COMPSE 2020, LNICST 359, pp. 143–154, 2021.
https://doi.org/10.1007/978-3-030-69839-3_10

specialties in general or specialty hospitals and has diagnostic imaging and laboratory support services. The third level provides specialized attention to greater complexity and combined with clinical and basic research activities. Teaching and research studies are also carried out here [2].

National Rehabilitation Institute Luis Guillermo Ibarra Ibarra (INR) is a third public hospital, whose scope of action includes the entire national territory and its main objective is scientific research in the field of health, the education and training of qualified human resources, and the provision of medical care services for a high specialty. The INR has three Surgical Unit (SU): Human Communication: Ophthalmology with three Operating Room (OR), Otolaryngology with three OR, Orthopedics with ten OR and CENIAQ (Center for National Specialization and Intervention for Attention to Burns) with two OR.

1.1 Literature Review

Quality in healthcare is a direct correlation between the level of improved health services and the desired health outcomes of individuals and populations. Quality improvement (QI) consists of systematic and continuous actions that lead to measurable improvement in health care services and the health status of targeted patient groups [3]. Tolga Taner and others have mentioned the criticism to a healthcare organization of patient satisfaction in long-term, to improve it, healthcare providers must focus on six attributes for a QI: security, efficiency, efficacy, focus on the person, equity and accessibility, opportunity, and affordability [4]. Professionals who work in healthcare must demonstrate these attributes with organizational culture and monitor these attributes as a crucial element of organization philosophy.

Lean. Looks for a way to improve and optimize the production system, trying to eliminate or reduce all activities that do not add value to the production process (waste or Muda). The waste is everything that consumes resources but does not create value [5]. Categories of waste include: Transportation, Inventory, Motion, Underrated skills, Waiting, Overproduction, Over-processing, and Defects. Lean framework means: Use the necessary resources and the minimum time to do just what needs to be done and when it needs to be done [5].

Six Sigma. Aims to improve by finding and eliminating the causes of mistakes and defects in business processes [6]. "Six Sigma quality" is a term generally used to indicate that a process is well controlled [7]. A five-step define-measure- analyze-improve-control (DMAIC) methodology is used where each step outlines distinct and key activities.

Lean Six Sigma. The basic strategy of Lean Six Sigma (LSS) is to use the Lean strategy first to eliminate waste and make processes profitable. The DMAIC strategy is used to reduce errors/defects in Lean optimized processes, either by improving or replacing them [8]. LSS is a fact-based improvement philosophy that values defect/error prevention over defect/error detection [7]. The integration of the LSS as a methodology of improving the process performance provides several benefits to the organizations [9]. Six Sigma has the power to save millions of dollars in healthcare by combining its key components with the major principles of Lean [8]. Programs like LSS provide healthcare organizations with a viable approach to not only reduce costs but also improve quality [10].

Barberato Henrique and Godinho Filho, analyzed three databases where they filtered search criteria related to the terms: Lean, Six Sigma, LSS and medical care, hospital, research. The researchers eliminated redundancies keeping 118 and obtaining important conclusions: LSS represents the 22.0% of the studies analyzed; The most widely area explored in healthcare is Emergency Department with 13.6%, Operating Theatre have just a 6.8%; Only 21 countries published 100% of the researchers analyzed in this paper [11], where Mexico was not found.

Healthcare system is not modeled as an industry system that analyzes and studies the processes for the creation of a product, it does not plan the inventories of parts in a factory, it does not create transportation networks for pieces supply. Health care service is a human task where a client/patient flows by a process where quality service is provided and is expected to be the best possible quality, and if it's possible, upgrade to a quality improvement above time. For this reason, it must be modeled in a systemic and detailed way, analyzing, and studying every detail. There are many studies about LSS in healthcare systems in different departments for QI but Black explored LSS and showed that these studies do not fully consider the complex social interactions that make processes to form in organizations like hospitals [12].

Medical Devices (MD) are used in the daily work of physicians, they use these technologies to generate a better diagnosis, give the greatest treatment, help successfully with patient's recovery, etc. Shah and Robinson mentioned that medical device technology has become a touchstone of enlightened practice [13], and the World Health Organization explained that is an important issue because users are the ultimate beneficiaries of developments [14]. A Biomedical Engineering team in a hospital oversees the safety and maintenance of MD in all its areas. But what happens if the MD fails? In the industry, when a machine does not work in the right way in a process where a product flow to a client, we have consequences as loss of client satisfaction, defects, delay time, waiting time, money loss, etc. Any failure could be solved and avoiding this represents a good point to inquire. But we must remember that healthcare systems are complex, that means we are taking care of people, so we work with the flow of a patient, a human living being, through his recovery or health keeping process. So, let us reflect which is one of the areas where would be more important or of extreme emergency to prevent failures in MD? In surgical Units, at OR physicians do procedures of extreme care and eliminate MD failures would be a great opportunity to help the satisfactory result of surgical procedures. So, we decided to look for the causes that produce MD failures at the different OR while surgery implementing LSS tools and methodologies looking forward to quality improvement.

Research done in developing countries is significantly small and the lack of evidence about LSS initiatives in Latin American countries is two important points exposed by Henrique and Filho. A group of Mexican researchers looked for the state of LSS practices and their implementation at Mexican hospitals even if they are not published in the literature. They applied a survey to 30 Mexican hospitals across six states, using 258 participants, from top managers down to front-line staff, selected by a random process. They found the penetration of LSS in the Mexican health system is represented by 16% of respondent's participation, being equally used in public versus private hospitals [15].

With the above, we are allowed to highlight the importance of research and development of research the implementation of LSS in quality improvement in healthcare systems and I quote Barberato Henrique and Godinho Filho: "There is an immediate need for research in this field that not only describes what tools were applied and what were the results obtained … there are still some dark and unexplored issues" [11].

The implementation of LSS in SU in Mexico is an area of study opportunity that will generate an important contribution to quality research in the complex Mexican healthcare system, leading us to innovative and improved studies and this research field in our country. Additionally, the academic impact of these investigation projects, in a country where is not developed yet and there is practically no existence of literature, is the fact that it is being developed and at the time it is published. Start to create Mexican LSS implementation bibliography, where the actual state is shown, barriers are explained, methodologies are exposed and conclusions are shared, we begin to open a way to grow not just in the number of articles, also in the quality improvement in our country. So, this type of research will start to be considered in Mexico, and all of Latin America, leading to new findings, and concrete conclusions, that would help us improving and encouraging these investigations. The objective of this research project is to implement LSS to identify and analyze the causes which produce failures in MD while surgery procedure in OR using the optimum tools, looking for quality improvement and applying three quality approaches: efficiency, efficacy, and security; and generate concrete conclusions about the analyzed and observed while the investigation project.

2 Methodology

QI process in the health field involves very important aspects: consider the healthcare organization as a system within a system of processes related to the guarantee of the quality of healthcare, understand and respect the expectations and quality requirements of the clinical efficacy of the patient/client, ensure that all staff in the healthcare organization work as a team to QI and collection and analysis of qualitative and quantitative data to monitor the quality of clinical effectiveness throughout the healthcare organization.

The regulatory framework of the NRI dictates that when an MD requires a service must be channeled through Biomedical Engineering Department (BED) and every action carried out on a medical device is recorded in a Biomedical Equipment Service Order (BESO), signed by the Department and the user area. The BESO must be registered in the SIAEM (Medical Equipment Administration Computer System). The BED has a calendar for preventive maintenance which is renovated every year. The activities of the Biomedical Engineer (BE) refer to any of the following activities, depending on the schedules or needs presented: Corrective maintenance, preventive maintenance, electrical safety tests, carry out service orders, training, and work with External Providers (EP).

We implemented the first three steps of the LSS using different tools to reach the elimination of waste and mistakes in the processes of preparation of MD in the Orthopedic and Human Communication SU. The tools used through the project development are shown in Table 1.

Table 1. LSS tools used in the project.

Step	Tool	Purpose
Define	5 s diagnosis	Measure quality performance and control with 5 s: Sort, Set in order, Shine, Standardize, Sustain
	Thread diagram	Identify waste in the engineer's work routine
	Interviews	Obtain information to generate a brainstorm. (surgeons, nursery team, BED team, and EP)
	Brainstorm	Identify the most commons problems with the MD
	Problem selection	Group the ideas of the brainstorm in the main ideas and obtained their frequency
	Pareto Chart I: *Brainstorm*	Calculate the cumulative frequency to build a Pareto Chart, identify the 20% vitals, and 80% trivial
	Pareto Chart II: *SIAEM*	Collect data from 2018 to March 2020 services done to the MD to build a Pareto Chart and identify the 20% vitals and 80% trivial
Measure	Value Stream Map (VSM)	Identify the flow of the patient through the process and to determine the Kaizen Outburst (KO), which shows waste
Analyze	Why? – Why?	Determine the causes of a problem, at each level of the diagram, the question why? is answered, until we reach the root of the problem

3 Analysis Proposal

3.1 Orthopedic Surgical Unit

Define

With all the tools before mentioned implemented, we selected the most significant data due to get closer to a real diagnosis, these ideas are exposed as follows.

5 s Diagnosis. The SU obtained "Formal Achievement" with a score of 63/120 which means 76%, like the point are not close to 90, the SU has not implemented yet the first 4 s.

Pareto Chart I: Brainstorm. In the Fig. 1 we can see that in the vital 20 are "Mistakes using MD" and with the same percentage "Damages to the MD while using it". The first one refers to the failures due to not knowing how does the MD works, therefore, not knowing how to use it properly, and the second refers to the existing carelessness when using it such as: dragging, hitting, throw cables, or parts, mistreating.

Pareto Chart II: SIAEM. The vital few reside in the "Steam Sterilizers", these are sheltered in the Sterilization Center and this does not affect directly while surgery, so we move on to the following percentage "Vital Sign Monitor", which has been replaced by new ones. So, the 20% range is discarded to decrease bias. Let's remember, the best tool is which provides us with the required information.

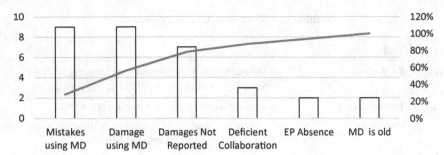

Fig. 1. The percentages obtained in the Pareto Chart I are: Mistakes using MD (28%), Damage using MD (28%), Damages nor Reported (22%), Deficient Collaboration between departments (9%), EP Absence (6%) and MD is old (6%).

Measure

From the last mains ideas, we connected them with the KO to realize a better interpretation of the problematic.

VSM. Considering the purpose of the project (identify the failures of MD in SU) we analyzed the processes carried out by the BE. There are 3 KO shown in Fig. 2: MD damages not reported to the BED, BE realizes this, it produces a delay in the preparation of the MD the next surgery, and sometimes these damages are not visible, consequently, the magnitude of the damage increases too; Frequent absence of the EP, MD is under a contract, which stipulates that an engineer from the supplier company will prepare this equipment before surgery. If EP is absent, the BE will have extra workload; Corrective Maintenance, If MD failure while surgery, Pareto Chart I show the causes of it.

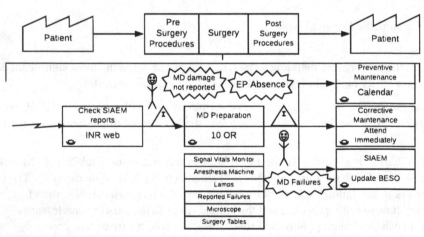

Fig. 2. At the beginning of the VSM, we can see the patient flow through the healthcare process. It is focused on the surgery process; it shows the flow of the BE through this process and the relation between the BE and MD.

Analyze

To finally define the problem and get to the exactly main causes of it, we dig into the resolutions given by the previous steps.

Why? -Why? The main cause provided by this technique is the non-attendance by the user to training and its consequences: from quality decrease to an economic point of view: expenditure in repairs. We analyzed a step behind, Lack of training, digging in this because it is important to explain the INR regulatory framework, which stipulates: Annually, a survey will be done to detect training needs, BED will establish with the Department Head the training needed and if a department of the hospital needs training, it must be solicited to the DEB, as soon as the need arises. So, the training service exists but it is not required, so the responsibility lies on the User (Fig. 3).

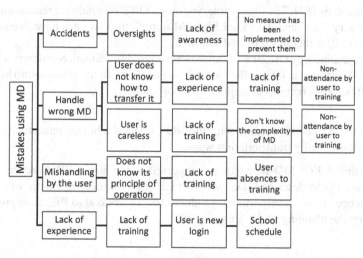

Fig. 3. Shows the main causes which are Non-attendance by the user to training.

3.2 Human Communication Surgical Unit

Define

The most significant data due to getting closer to a real diagnosis were given by the threading diagram and Pareto Charts.

5 s Diagnosis. The SU obtained "Formal Achievement" with a score of 67/120 which means 80%.

Thread Diagram. We found transportation waste because of the planning of the SU.

Pareto Chart I: Brainstorm. The vital problem is the "Area Planning", which is discarded so, the next category is the "Mistakes while using MD", this is analyzed further. We can see this result in Fig. 4.

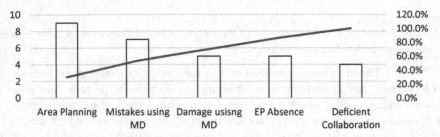

Fig. 4. The percentages obtained in the Pareto Chart I are: Area Planning (30%), Mistakes using MD (23.3%), Damages using MD (16.7%), EP Absence (16.7%), and Deficient Collaboration between departments (13.3%).

Pareto Chart II: SIAEM. The Otorhinolaryngology OR 20% vitals are represented by the "Electrosurgery Unit" and the "Vital Signs Monitor", the last ones have been replaced in December 2019, therefore, were discarded.

The Ophthalmology OR 20% of failures are caused by "Steam Sterilizers". For both areas, the MD is found in OR, so the biomedical engineer can incorporate into his routine checking it before surgery, preventing them from failing.

Measure

We connected the last main ideas with the KO to obtain a bigger interpretation of the problematic, especially transportation waste.

VSM. We find 5 KO: MD damages not reported to the BED, EP Absence and MD Failures haven been described; Delay of the EP (EP Absence) in charge of preparing the microscope and the transportation produces too a workload to BE; Transport Waste, produced by the planning of the area (Fig. 5).

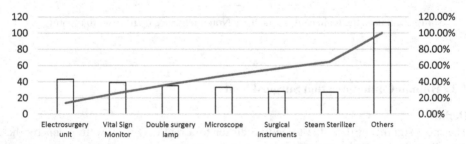

Fig. 5. The percentages obtained in the Pareto Chart II (Otorhinolaryngology SU) are Electrosurgery unit (13.5%), Vital Sign Monitor (12.6%), Double surgery lamp (11.01%), Microscope (10.38%), Surgical instruments (8.81%), Steam Sterilizer (8.49%) and Others (35.53%).

Analyze

We dig and compare the main ideas reached to finally define the problem and to know exactly the main causes of the problem. It must be considered that the poor planning and design of the area and its resolution is not included in the project limitations (Fig. 6).

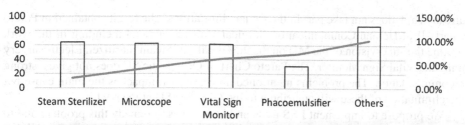

Fig. 6. The percentages obtained in the Pareto Chart II (Ophthalmology OR) are: Steam Sterilizer (20.98%), Microscope (20.33%), Vital Signal Monitor (20.00%), Phacoemulsifier (10.16%), and Others (28.52%).

Why? -Why? Considering that the problem to be analyzed is "Mistakes while using MD", the causes converge to the same root cause in the first Why? - Why? diagram.

4 Results

During the project development, we identified the mistakes and wastes that cause MD failures while surgery procedures at the INR's SU. The main cause is the lack of training by the user, and this main cause was analyzed. The analysis leads us to identify the real main cause which is the non-assistance to training and that this training are also not required by the user. The failures of the MD in Orthopedics and Human Communication SU, would be solved with the increase in the number of training provided with the complete assistance of the user (Fig. 7).

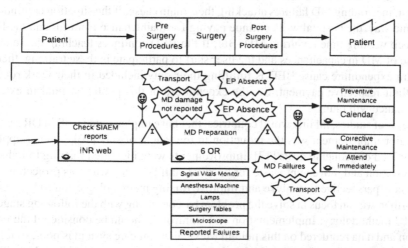

Fig. 7. At the beginning of the VSM, we can see the patient flow through the healthcare process. It is focused on the surgery process; it shows the flow of the BE through this process and the relation between the BE and MD. It shows 6 KO.

The absence of the EP should be deal with by the provider to set and re-structure the contract and avoid the work overload to the BE. Transportation waste, like it has been already said, does not take part in the project limitations. The results obtained in Pareto Charts II at Human Communication Surgical Unit recommend including in the work routine the supervision of the MD on the 20% vitals, as Steam Sterilizer, Electrosurgery unit, and Vital Sign Monitor. The Pareto Chart of Orthopedic SU does not give a strong recommendation. The problems mentioned above do not impact as the main cause but the elimination of these will contribute to the QI in the SU at the NRI.

We propose to implement LSS tools and techniques to remedy this problem and to reach QI in the hospital. We also recommend to strength the training given: explaining the care importance; showing how does the MD work to help the user area to understand the operating principle basis, so they would manipulate it in the right way; motivate users to be part of this training. If the previous recommendations are taken, the INR will eliminate MD failures at SU and get a QI achievement.

5   Conclusions

As the first three stages of DMAIC have been implemented, and the real main cause that produces MD failures at SU of the INR has been identifying, the lack of training, and the non-participation of the user on it. Once we conclude it, we checked the regulations from the hospital, where we realized two crucial points: the capacitance that is requested has a low number of participants and the lack of more training it's because the user area does not request them. We strongly recommend starting participating in training and understanding the importance of knowing the function of MD to avoid its failures while surgery, prevent it malfunction and decreasing the number of corrective maintenances.

Above its essential to understand the economic impact, we are studying a public hospital, in avoiding MD failures attacking their main cause. If the situation continues in the same way, the hospital will continue paying for maintenance from EP and the BED will keep wasting time repairing MD. But, If the BED continues teaching the function and use of MD in capacitances and the user start to participate in these training, there is no extra expenditure cause BED is fulfilling their duty included in their work routine, so in their respective payment. So, the expenditure of this public hospital in external maintenance will plunge.

Major of studies, inf first world countries, that have implemented LSS in OR reached like major improvement was the reduction in the length of stay [16], another application focused on reducing costs [17], improvements were identified relating to reducing transportation and movement waste for hospital staff [18]. So, with this project, we can give a new perspective to analyze and improve quality methodologies on SU.

Further, we can focus in solve the problem by continuing with the following stages of DMAIC methodology: Implementation and Control. It should be considered the investigation and data reordered on this field in Mexican healthcare system is poor, so it must be registered every step and detail of the research, project, or investigation done. Then, the work registrations could be used in other research as a starting point or comparative way.

So, for a further project, we can work with Implementation by applying the solutions to the problem that has been identified. We should consider the limitations and the situations that could occur while this: opposition to change the way it has been worked through the years, close minds, the lack of evidence (we must remember that in Mexico all the healthcare work is done basis on evidence), change resistance, etc. It would be essential to compare the situation before and after the performance of this stage, and from this comparison determined the benefits and results of implementing quality methodologies.

For the Control stage, we can perform other investigation projects. After the implementation stage, we should look for keeping the achievements that have been acquired. In the final DMAIC stage, we want to standardize the new work routines as the natural way of performing the duties. We can speculate that it would be harder this stage (Control) than the previous one (Implementation). This is predicted because it is easier to perform new routines for a given time than integrate a new way to do something like the usual routine (longer period). When you propose to someone to work in a different way than the person has always done, it will always bring resistance, and with more reason, if it is a permanent change.

The following projects of this investigation would be registered in the right way to bring new data and conclusions in this field. We expect this new research to help and promote the investigation about QI in Mexican healthcare system, and lead to concrete the fundaments of it.

The National Association of Faculties and Schools of Engineering suggested the design of a society that meets new needs in the field of health and highlighted the requirements of engineering to face it, so medical technology develops holistic and complex intervention systems, in which engineering will surely also play an important role [19]. So as Mexican quality healthcare investigations, we contribute helping with the beginning of the writing literature about LSS implementation in Mexican Healthcare Systems and Latin-American countries. The given conclusions will help another research as a pillar or argument in their new investigation projects, this continuous practice would lead to improving the number of research, implementation, literature but more important, quality in Mexican healthcare system.

Acknowledgment. This research was supported by National Autonomous University of Mexico (UNAM), PAPIIT IA105220 Optimización en la Logística Hospitalaria.

References

1. Gómez Dantés, O., Sesma, S., Becerril, V., Knaul, F., Arreola, H., Frenk, J.: Sistema de salud de México. Salud Pública de México (58) (2011)
2. Rea Ruanova, B.: Los tres niveles de salud. https://www.meditips.com/los-tres-niveles-atencion-salud/
3. U. S. Department of Health and Human Services Health Resources and Services Administration: Quality Improvement (2011). https://www.hrsa.gov/sites/default/files/quality/toolbox/508pdfs/qualityimprovement.pdf
4. Tolga-Taner, M., Sezen, B., Antony, J.: An overview of six sigma applications in healthcare industry. Int. J. Health Care Qual. Assur. **20**(4), 329–340 (2007)
5. Womack, J.P., Roos, D., Jones, D.: The Machine That Changed the World/Lean Thinking. Free Press, NY (2007)

6. Ramu, G.: The Certified Six Sigma Yellow Belt Handbook, 1st edn. American Society for Quality, Milwaukee (2017)
7. American Society of Quality: What is Six Sigma? https://asq.org/quality-resources/six-sigma
8. Wickramasinghe, N., Al-Hakim, L., Gonzalez, Ch., Tan, J.: Lean Thinking for Healthcare. Springer, Chicago (2014)
9. de Freitas, J., Costa, H.: Impacts of Lean Six Sigma over organizational sustainability. Int. J. Lean Six Sigma (8), 89–108 (2017)
10. Foster, T.J.: Does Six Sigma improve performance? Qual. Manage. J. **14**(4), 7–20 (2007)
11. Barberato Henrique, D., Godinho Filho, M.: A systematic literature review of empirical research in Lean and Six Sigma in healthcare. Total Qual. Manage. Bus. Excellence **31**, 1–21 (2018)
12. Black, J.: Transforming the patient care environment with Lean Six Sigma and realistic evaluation. J. Healthc. Qual. **31**(3), 29–35 (2009)
13. Shah, S., Robinson, I.: User involvement in medical device technology development and assessment: a structured literature review. Int. J. Health Care Qual. Assur. **6**(19), 500–515 (2006)
14. Organization, W.H.: Medical Device Regulations: Global Overview and Guiding Principles. de World Health Organization, Geneva (2003)
15. Peimbert-García, R.E., et al.: Assessing the state of lean and six sigma practices in healthcare in Mexico. Emerald Publishing Limited **32**(4), 664–662 (2019)
16. Honda, A.C., Bernardo, M.: How Lean Six Sigma principles improve hospital performance. Qual. Manage. J. **25**(2), 70–82 (2018)
17. Gayed, B., Black, J.S., Daggy, I., Munshi, A.: Redesigning a joint replacement program using Lean Six Sigma in a Veterans affairs hospital. JAMA Surg. **148**(11), 1050–1056 (2013)
18. Aakre, K.T., Valley, T.B., O'Connor, M.K.: Quality initiatives: improving patient flow for a bone densitometry practice: results from a Mayo Clinic radiology quality initiative. Radiographics **30**(2), 309–315 (2010)
19. National Association of Faculties and Schools of Engineering (ANFEI), Engineering Mexico 2030: Future Scenarios. ANFEI, pp. 115–137. Mexico. ANFEI (2003)
20. Glasgow, J., Scott-Caziewell, J., Kaboli, P.: Guiding inpatient quality improvement: a systematic review of Lean and Six Sigma. Joint Comm. J. Qual. Patient Saf. **36**(12), 533-AP5 (2010)

Applied Optimization

MTGWA: A Multithreaded Gray Wolf Algorithm with Strategies Based on Simulated Annealing and Genetic Algorithms

Felix Martinez-Rios[1]([✉]) [iD], Alfonso Murillo-Suarez[1] [iD],
Cesar Raul Garcia-Jacas[2] [iD], and Juan Manuel Guerrero-Valadez[1] [iD]

[1] Facutad de Ingeniería, Universidad Panamericana, Mexico City, Mexico
{felix.martinez,alfonso.murillosuarez,
juanmanuel.guerrerovaladez}@up.edu.mx
[2] Departamento de Ciencias de la Computación, CICESE,
Ensenada, Baja California, Mexico
cesarrjacas1985@gmail.com

Abstract. In this paper, we present an improvement of the Gray Wolf algorithm (GWO) based on a multi-threaded implementation of the original algorithm. The paper demonstrates how to combine the solutions obtained in each of the threads to achieve a final solution closer to the absolute minimum or even equal to it. To properly combine the solutions of each of the threads of execution, we use strategies based on simulated annealing and genetic algorithms. Also, we show the results obtained for twenty-nine functions: unimodal, multimodal, fixed dimension and composite functions. Experiments show that our proposed improves the results of the original algorithm.

Keywords: Nature-inspired algorithm · Optimization ·
Multi-threaded execution · Optimization techniques · Metaheuristics ·
Gray Wolf algorithm

1 Introduction

Metaheuristic optimization algorithms have developed impressively in the last two decades. Some of these, such as Artificial Bee Colony (ABC) [9,10,31], Ant Colony Optimization (ACO) [4,24,25], Bat-Inspired Algorithm (BAT) [1,19,29], Particle Swarm Optimization (PSO) [5,8,22], have had great repercussions among scientists from different fields. Metaheuristics have become popular methods for solving problems for four main reasons: simplicity, flexibility, derivation-free mechanism and optimal local avoidance [12].

The metaheuristics are quite simple and have been mostly inspired by concepts related to physical phenomena, natural phenomena or animal behaviors in nature. This simplicity allows metaheuristics to be applied to different problems

© ICST Institute for Computer Sciences, Social Informatics and Telecommunications Engineering 2021
Published by Springer Nature Switzerland AG 2021. All Rights Reserved
J. A. Marmolejo-Saucedo et al. (Eds.): COMPSE 2020, LNICST 359, pp. 157–172, 2021.
https://doi.org/10.1007/978-3-030-69839-3_11

without special changes in the structure of the algorithm. Also, most meta-heuristics are free of derivation because, unlike gradient-based optimization approaches, metaheuristics optimizes the problems stochastically, the process begins with random solutions which are modified with the metaheuristic in the search space to find the optimum. Finally, metaheuristics have superior capabilities to avoid local optimum. Compared to conventional optimization techniques because due to the stochastic nature of metaheuristics, it allows them to avoid local solutions [16,30].

The metaheuristic algorithms can be divided into two main classes: those based on a single solution (for example, Simulated Annealing [6,11,13]) and those based on populations (for example, Firefly algorithm [3,17,26]). In the single solution based search process, start with a candidate solution. This unique candidate solution then improves throughout the iterations. The population-based metaheuristics use a set of random initial solutions called population, and are improved for the iterations. Population-based metaheuristics have some advantages over single solution metaheuristics. Multiple candidate solutions share information about the search space that provokes in sudden leaps towards more promising values; these multiple candidate solutions mutually cooperate to avoid optimal solutions locally. Finally, population-based metaheuristics generally have a higher and better search space exploration compared to algorithms based on individual solutions [2,7,30].

One of the most exciting branches of population-based metaheuristics is swarm intelligence (SI). SI algorithms are easy to implement. A common feature is the division of the search process into two phases: exploration and exploitation. The exploration phase refers to the research process of the promising areas of the search space. Exploitation refers to the search capacity in the promising regions obtained in the exploration phase. Find a proper balance between these two phases is considered a difficult task due to the stochastic nature of metaheuristics [15,21].

2   Gray Wolf Algorithm

Gray wolves are considered top predators of the food chain. Gray wolves mostly prefer to live in a herd of size with 5 to 12 wolves on average. These herds have a rigorous dominant social hierarchy. The leaders are male and female called alphas and are responsible for making decisions about hunting, resting places, etc. The pack obeys the decisions of the alpha wolf. The second level in the gray wolf hierarchy is beta. The betas are subordinate wolves that help the alpha in decision making or other activities. The beta wolf respects the alpha but gives orders to the lower level. The lesser gray wolf is omega. It may seem that omega is not an important individual in the group, but it has been observed that they maintain the structure of domination and care of the young. If a wolf is not alpha, neither beta nor omega, it is called delta, and they have functions of scouts and sentries.

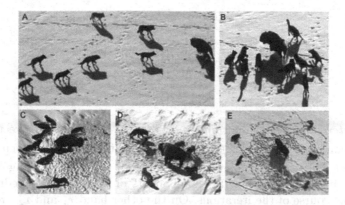

Fig. 1. Typical behaviors of wolf hunting in Yellowstone National Park. (A) Approach, track, and persecution of the prey. (B - D) Persecution, harassment and surrounding maneuver. (E) Wolves at the end of the hunt in the last configuration that approximates a regular polygon [20].

In addition to the social hierarchy of wolves mentioned above, group hunting is another interesting social behavior of gray wolves. According to Muro et al. [20], the main phases of the gray wolf hunt are:

1. Tracking, chasing, and approaching the dam.
2. Pursue, surround, and harass the dam until it stops.
3. The movement to surround it.
4. Attack on the prey.

GWO algorithm [18,27,28] models this technique of hunting and social hierarchy to perform the optimization. In Fig. 1, we can see real examples of these stages.

To model the social hierarchy of wolves, we consider that the alpha wolf (X_α) is the one in the position with the lowest value of the function to optimize in each iteration of the algorithm. Equally, the second and third-best solutions are named beta wolf (X_β) and delta wolf (X_α), respectively. As mentioned earlier, gray wolves surround their prey during hunting and to model this behavior the following equations are proposed:

$$\vec{D} = \left| \vec{C} * \vec{X_p}(iter) - \vec{X_i}(iter) \right| \tag{1}$$

$$\vec{X}(iter + 1) = \vec{X_p}(iter) - \vec{A} * \vec{D} \tag{2}$$

$$\vec{D_\alpha} = \left| \vec{C_1} * \vec{X_\alpha} - \vec{X_i} \right|$$

$$\vec{D_\beta} = \left| \vec{C_1} * \vec{X_\beta} - \vec{X_i} \right| \tag{3}$$

$$\vec{D_\delta} = \left| \vec{C_1} * \vec{X_\delta} - \vec{X_i} \right|$$

$$\vec{A} = 2\,\vec{a}\,\vec{r_1} - \vec{a} \tag{4}$$

$$\vec{a} = 2 - 2\frac{iteration}{MaxIterations} \tag{5}$$

$$\vec{C} = 2\vec{r_2} \tag{6}$$

where *iter* indicates the current iteration, $\vec{X_p}$ is the position vector of the prey (position of the alpha wolf), and $\vec{X_i}$ indicates the position of each gray wolf in the group. The vectors $\vec{A}$ and $\vec{D}$ are calculated with the following equations:

In Eq. 5 it can be seen how the components of $\vec{a}$ are linearly reduced from 2 to 0 in the course of the iterations. On the other hand $\vec{r_1}$ and $\vec{r_2}$ are random vectors in the interval $[0, 1)$.

Gray wolves can recognize the location of the prey and surround it, the alpha wolf guides this process and the beta wolf and delta have a better idea of the position of the prey than the rest of the group. To simulate the above, we keep the three best positions (alpha, beta and, delta wolves respectively) regarding the value of the function we are optimizing. The remaining wolves update their positions using the following equations:

$$\begin{aligned} \vec{X_1} &= \vec{X_\alpha} - \vec{A_1} * \vec{D_\alpha} \\ \vec{X_2} &= \vec{X_\beta} - \vec{A_2} * \vec{D_\beta} \\ \vec{X_3} &= \vec{X_\delta} - \vec{A_3} * \vec{D_\delta} \end{aligned} \tag{7}$$

$$\vec{X}(iter + 1) = \frac{\vec{X_1}(iter) + \vec{X_2}(iter) + \vec{X_3}(iter)}{3} \tag{8}$$

The pseudocode of the GWO algorithm is presented in Algorithm 1. Random parameters $\vec{A}$ and $\vec{C}$ help the candidate solutions to have hyper-spheres with different random radii for the search space exploration process. The balance between exploration and exploitation is guaranteed by the values of $\vec{a}$ and $\vec{A}$, which allow the algorithm a smooth transition between smooth exploration exploitation.

The multi-threaded implementation of the Gray Wolf Algorithm shown in Algorithm 1 starts initializing six parameters:

1. **N_GW** number of Gray Wolf by each thread τ in P.
2. **P** value that indicates how many iterations of each thread τ will execute before the implementation of the selected crossover technique.
3. **MaxIter** indicates the total number of iterations of the Gray Wolf Algorithm that each thread is going to execute.
4. **S**best is the best solution obtained.

Algorithm 1: Pseudocode of the Gray Wolf Algorithm (GWO).

Data: n,MaxIterations
Result: Function fitness and position

1 **begin**
2   Initialize the Gray Wolf population $W = w_i(i = 1, 2, ..., n)$
3   Calculate $\overrightarrow{A}$, $\overrightarrow{a}$, and $\overrightarrow{C}$ using Eqs. 4, 5, and 6
4   Calculate the fitness for each wolf w_i
5   X_α = the best wolf agent
6   X_β = the second best wolf agent
7   X_δ = the third best wolf agent
8    $iter = 1$
9   **while** $iter \leq MaxIterations$ **do**
10   **foreach** $wolf\ w_i\ from\ W\ population$ **do**
11   Update X_i position of w_i using Eq. 8
12   **end**
13   Update $\overrightarrow{A}$, $\overrightarrow{a}$, and $\overrightarrow{C}$ using Eqs. 4, 5, and 6
14   Calculate the fitness for each wolf w_i
15   Update X_α = the best wolf agent
16   Update X_β = the second best wolf agent
17   Update X_δ = the third best wolf agent
18   **end**
19   Return the best solution X_α and function fitness
20 **end**

The multithreaded implementation of GWA executes independent versions of Algorithm 1 on each thread, as shown in Algorithm 2 on line 7, until the number of iterations in each thread reaches the cut-off value P. Once the cutoff value is reached, all threads return the solution reached S_τ^{best}, and the best of all solutions S^{best} is obtained (lines 9 to 11 Algorithm 2), once this is done, the crossover techniques are executed. In the experiments for this work, four crossover techniques were implemented.

- **To the best(TB):** This cross method takes the thread with the best solution S^{best} and copies the values obtained for all other threads.
- **Annealing to the best (ATB):** Similar to the simulated Annealing algorithm [6], in this ease, the best solution obtained S^{best} is copied to the rest of the threads when the following condition is met: [9]:

$$rand\,[0,1) \leq exp\left(-\frac{1}{\log\left(\frac{MaxIter}{t}\right)}\right) \qquad (9)$$

$$foreach\ \tau\ in\ P$$
$$if\ \tau \neq \tau_{best}$$
$$for\ i\ =\ 1\ to\ pos \qquad (10)$$
$$S_\tau(i) = S^{best}(i)$$

- **Genetic with the best (GTB):** This method is inspired by the procedures of the genetic algorithm [13]. A random number $pos = rand(1, dimension)$ is selected and, the first pos values of the best solution are combined with the results of each of the remaining threads as:
- **Annealing genetic with the best (AGTB):** This method combines the previous two (Annealing to best and Genetic whit the best) if Eq. 9 is true, we execute the combination of the best solution $S^{best}(i)$ with the remaining threads using the Eq. 10.

Algorithm 2: MTGWA: Multi-threaded implementation of Gray Wolf Algorithm.

    Data: N_GW, P, $MaxIter$, S^{best}
    Result: S^{best}

1 **begin**
2 | **foreach** τ *in* Γ **do**
3 | | Initialize τ with $n = N\_GW$, $MaxIterations = P$
4 | **end**
5 | $t \leftarrow 0$
6 | **while** $t \leq MaxIter$ **do**
7 | | **foreach** τ *in* Γ **do**
8 | | | Execute GWA (Algorith 1) in τ for P iterations
9 | | | $S_\tau^{best} \leftarrow$ best solution obtained in τ
10 | | | **if** S_τ^{best} *is better than* S^{best} **then**
11 | | | | $S^{best} \leftarrow S_\tau^{best}$
12 | | | **end**
13 | | **end**
14 | | **foreach** τ *in* Γ **do**
15 | | | Execute thread-crossover technique
16 | | **end**
17 | | $t \leftarrow t + P$
18 | **end**
19 | Return S^{best}
20 **end**

In Fig. 2 we see how Algorithm 2 works. K threads of the GWO algorithm are executed; each one improves its solution S_i. When the threads reach iteration P, and each one returns its best solution. For example, in iteration P, suppose that the best solution was obtained by thread 3 (box red), then in generation $P + 1$ all the wires continue to run based on the initial solution obtained by thread 3 and it is constructed using one of the four crossover methods explained above.

As seen in Fig. 2, the execution of the threads continues until the generations reach the next $2P$ value cut, and for example in this case, the best result is reached by thread 2. Then the process of the solution combination is repeated and the algorithm continues until the last generation M.

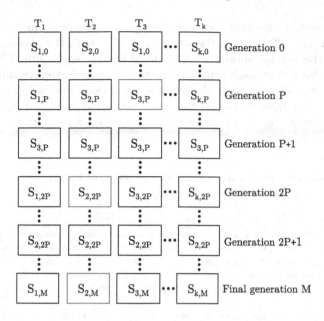

Fig. 2. Operation of the multithreaded implementation of the Gray Wolves algorithm. k is the number og threads, M is the maximum number of iterations and P is the cutoff value. (Color figure online)

3   Experiments

In this section, different experiments are carried out to tune the parameters used in Algorithm 2. The parameters we need to tune are the value of the cut generation P and the number of threads that will be used. We will use the same functions as Mirjalili et al. to compare our results with those previously obtained [18]. The benchmark function used for the experiments is shown in Tables 3, 4, 5, and 6 obtained from [14]. For all the experiments, we used a swarm with 30 gray wolves. All experiments were executed in a Dell Inspiron 7472 laptop, with Intel Core i7-8550U, with Microsoft's Windows 10 Home OS, and 16 GB of RAM. The algorithm was developed in C#.

To tune the algorithm parameters, we will execute it 30 times with each of the 13 selected multimodal and unimodal functions. In Table 1, we can see the results of the algorithm for different cut-off values P. With these results and taking into account the cut-off value with which our algorithm obtained the lowest value of the objective function, we can select $P = 100$ (making an average weighted of the P values for which the lowest optimization value was obtained).

Now with the value of $P = 100$, we will execute the algorithm modifying the number of threads that are used. Table 2 shows the results of the algorithm executions with 2 threads up to 10 threads.

With the results obtained and shown in Table 2, we performed a check with the Wilcoxon test [23] between the results obtained with the original algorithm and each of the results obtained with our MTGWA algorithm. This analysis showed that from 6 threads, our algorithm achieved better results than the original. We also observed that the average execution time was 5 s for each of the functions, but from 9 threads the execution time increased by 20%. With the previous results, we will execute the four crossover variants for 6, 7, and 8 threads.

Table 1. Results of experiments to tune the cut-off value P. The best value obtained for each function appears in bold.

Id	GWO	50	100	150	200	250	300	350	400	450
f1	6.59E-28	**9.93E-29**	1.06E-28	1.62E-28	1.86E-28	3.93E-28	5.04E-28	2.08E-28	6.28E-28	6.04E-28
f2	7.18E-17	**2.40E-17**	3.19E-17	5.06E-17	5.73E-17	3.87E-17	4.13E-17	5.01E-17	5.73E-17	3.96E-17
f3	3.29E-06	**1.10E-26**	5.15E-26	3.83E-26	3.96E-26	2.75E-26	5.37E-26	1.90E-26	7.67E-26	6.74E-26
f4	5.61E-07	**1.16E-08**	1.52E-08	1.90E-08	2.80E-08	2.35E-08	3.14E-08	2.58E-08	2.95E-08	2.51E-08
f5	26.81	26.48	26.61	26.26	26.77175	**26.33**	26.67	26.76	26.60	26.47
f6	0.816	0	0	0	0	0	0	0	0	0
f7	0.00221	0.00103	0.00102	**0.00145**	0.00148	0.00158	0.00113	0.00127	0.00140	0.00179
f8	**−6123**	−3341	−3955	−4339	−4542	−5028	−5066	−5196	−5281	−5201
f9	0.310	0.480	0.342	1.33	0.432	**0.225**	0.794	0.704	0.552	0.799
f10	1.06E-13	**1.07E-14**	7.39E-14	7.96E-14	7.36E-14	7.39E-14	8.39E-14	8.25E-14	7.93E-14	2.28E-14
f11	0.00448	0.00115	0.00270	0.00122	0.00121	0	0	0	0	0
f12	0.0534	0.0418	0.0402	**0.0244**	0.0280	0.0334	0.0356	0.0415	0.0286	0.0266
f13	0.654464	0.430	0.431	0.480	**0.429**	0.421	0.557	0.440	0.480	0.606

Table 2. Results of executions with $P = 100$ and the number of threads between 2 and 10.

Id	GWO	2	3	4	5	6	7	8	9	10
f1	6.59E-28	1.08E-28	5.67E-29	2.56E-29	5.46E-29	2.62E-29	1.97E-29	1.76E-29	1.08E-29	1.02E-29
f2	7.18E-17	3.21E-17	1.68E-17	1.86E-17	1.67E-17	8.87E-18	1.08E-17	1.41E-17	1.25E-17	9.77E-18
f3	3.29E-06	1.53E-26	1.48E-26	9.59E-27	5.28E-27	4.68E-27	2.94E-27	1.37E-27	2.13E-27	1.68E-27
f4	5.61E-07	2.34E-08	1.68E-08	1.38E-08	6.76E-09	5.66E-09	4.63E-09	4.31E-09	4.34E-09	3.38E-09
f5	26.81	26.87	26.57	26.40	26.62	26.13	26.34	26.08	26.09	26.51
f6	0.81658	0	0	0	0	0	0	0	0	0
f7	0.00221	0.00154	0.00064	0	0	0	0	0	0	0
f8	−6123	−3837	−4376	−4293	−4381	−4423	−4394	−4543	−4521	−4444
f9	3.11E-01	5.06E-01	6.04E-15	4.26E-15	3.55E-16	0	0	0	0	3.55E-16
f10	1.06E-13	5.48E-14	6.26E-14	6.05E-14	4.31E-14	4.49E-14	2.50E-14	4.81E-14	4.13E-14	2.82E-14
f11	0.00449	0.00088	0	0	0	0	0	0	0	0
f12	0.05344	0.03485	0.01971	0.02850	0.02111	0.01842	0.02185	0.01538	0.01905	0.01377
f13	0.65446	0.45689	0.47354	0.46292	0.37474	0.32217	0.31358	0.34517	0.21400	0.30800

Table 3. Unimodal benchmark functions.

f	Function	Mathematical Equation	Dimensions	Search space	Minimum
$f1$	Sphere	$f(x) = \sum\limits_{i=1}^{d} x_i^2$	30	$x_i \epsilon\,[-100, 100]$	$f(x) = 0$
$f2$	Schwefel 2.22	$f(x) = \sum\limits_{i=1}^{d} |x_i| + \prod\limits_{i=1}^{d} |x_i|$	30	$x_i \epsilon\,[-10, 10]$	$f(x) = 0$
$f3$	Rotated Hyperellipsoid	$f(x) = \sum\limits_{i=1}^{d} \left(\sum\limits_{j=1}^{i} x_j \right)^2$	30	$x_i \epsilon\,[-100, 100]$	$f(x) = 0$
$f4$	Schwefel 2.21	$f(x) = \max\limits_{i=1,\ldots,d} |x_i|$	30	$x_i \epsilon\,[-10, 10]$	$f(x) = 0$
$f5$	Rosenbrock	$f(x) = \sum\limits_{i=1}^{d} \left[100\left(x_{i+1} - x_i^2\right)^2 + (x_i - 1)^2 \right]$	30	$x_i \epsilon\,[-30, 30]$	$f(x) = 0$
$f6$	Step 2	$f(x) = \sum\limits_{i=1}^{d} \lfloor x_i + 0.5 \rfloor^2$	30	$x_i \epsilon\,[-100, 100]$	∞ and $f(x) = 0$
$f7$	Quartic with noise	$f(x) = \sum\limits_{i=1}^{d} ix_i^2 + random\,[0, 1]$	30	$x_i \epsilon\,[-1.28, 1.28]$	$f(x) = 0 + random\,[0, 1]$

Table 4. Multimodal benchmark functions.

f	Function	Mathematical Equation	Dimensions	Search space	Minimum
$f8$	Schwefel	$f(x) = 418.9829d - \sum\limits_{i=1}^{d} x_i \sin\left(\sqrt{|x_i|}\right)$	30	$x_i \epsilon\,[-500, 500]$	$f(x) = 0$
$f9$	Rastrigin	$f(x) = \sum\limits_{i=1}^{d} \left[x_i^2 - 10\cos\left(2\pi x_i\right) + 10 \right]$	30	$x_i \epsilon\,[-5.12, 5.12]$	$f(x) = 0$
$f10$	Ackley 1	$f(x) = -20\exp\left(-0.2\sqrt{\frac{1}{d}\sum\limits_{i=1}^{d} x_i^2}\right) - \exp\left(\frac{1}{d}\sum\limits_{i=1}^{d}\cos\left(2\pi x_i\right)\right) + 20 + \exp(1)$	30	$x_i \epsilon\,[-32, 32]$	$f(x) = 0$
$f11$	Griewank	$f(x) = \sum\limits_{i=1}^{d} \frac{x_i^2}{4000} - \prod\limits_{i=1}^{d}\cos\left(\frac{x_i}{\sqrt{i}}\right) + 1$	30	$x_i \epsilon\,[-600, 600]$	$f(x) = 0$
$f12$	Generalized Penalized 1	$F(x) = \frac{\pi}{d}\left\{ 10\sin^2\left(\pi y_1\right) + \sum\limits_{i=1}^{d-1}\left(y_i - 1\right)^2\left[1 + 10\sin^2\left(\pi y_{i+1}\right)\right] + (y_n - 1)^2 \right\}$ $+ \sum\limits_{i=1}^{d} u\left(x_i, a, k, m\right), where$ $y_i = 1 + \frac{1}{4}\left(x_i + 1\right), u\left(x_i, a, k, m\right) = \begin{cases} K\left(x_i - a\right)^m & x_i > a \\ 0 & -a \leq x_i \leq a \\ k\left(-x_i - a\right)^m & x_i < -a \end{cases}$ $a = 10, k = 100, m = 4$	30	$x_i \epsilon\,[-50, 50]$	$f(x) = 0$
$f13$	Generalized Penalized 2	$f(x) = 0.1\left\{ \sin^2\left(3\pi x_1\right) + \sum\limits_{i=1}^{d-1}\left(x_i - 1\right)^2\left[1 + \sin^2\left(3\pi x_{i+1}\right)\right] + (x_d - 1)^2\left[1 + \sin^2\left(2\pi x_d\right)\right] \right\}$ $+ \sum\limits_{i=1}^{d} u\left(x_i, a, k, m\right), where$ $u\left(x_i, a, k, m\right) = \begin{cases} K\left(x_i - a\right)^m & x_i > a \\ 0 & -a \leq x_i \leq a \\ k\left(-x_i - a\right)^m & x_i < -a \end{cases}$ $a = 5, k = 100, m = 4$	30	$x_i \epsilon\,[-50, 50]$	$f(x) = 0$

Tables 4 shows the results of the final experiments of our algorithm. For unimodal functions, we see that better results were obtained in all functions, even in functions $f6$ and $f7$, the exact minimum 0 was obtained. Experiments with multimodal functions also showed better results for our algorithm, although the expected minimum value was not reached in function $f8$. For multimodal functions of fixed dimension, the results reached the minimum expected values except in three functions $f20$, $f21$ and $f23$. The executions with the composite functions showed that our algorithm was better in 4 functions of the 6 tested (Tables 7, 8 and 9).

Table 5. Multimodal fixed-dimension benchmark functions.

f	Function	Mathematical Equation	Dimensions	Search space	Minimum
$f14$	Shekel's Foxhole	$f(x) = \left[\frac{1}{500} + \sum\limits_{j=1}^{25} \frac{1}{j + \sum\limits_{i=1}^{2}(x_i - a_{i,j})^6} \right]^{-1}$, where $a_{i,j} = \begin{pmatrix} -32 & -16 & 0 & 16 & 32 & -32 & 0 & 16 & 32 \\ -32 & -32 & -32 & -32 & -32 & -16 & \dots & 32 & 32 & 32 \end{pmatrix}$	2	$x_i \epsilon [-65.536, 65.536]$	$f(x) = 0.9980038377$
$f15$	Kowalik	$f(x) = \sum\limits_{i=1}^{10} \left[a_i - \frac{x_1(b_i^2 + b_i x_2)}{b_i^2 + b_i x_3 + x_4} \right]^2$, where $a = [0.1957, 0.1947, 0.1735, 0.16, 0.0844, 0.0627, 0.0456, 0.0342, 0.0323, 0.0235, 0.0246]$ $b = [4, 2, 1, 0.5, 0.25, 1/6, 0.125, 0.1, 1/12, 1/14, 0.0625]$	4	$x_i \epsilon [-5, 5]$	$f(x) = 0.00030748610$
$f16$	Six Hump Camel	$f(x) = \left(4 - 2.1 x_1^2 + \frac{x_1^4}{3} \right) x_1^2 + x_1 x_2 + (-4 + 4 x_2^2) x_2^2$	2	$x_i \epsilon [-5, 5]$	$f(x) = -1.0316285$
$f17$	Branin No. 1	$f(x) = \left(x_2 - \frac{5.1 x_1^2}{4\pi^2} + \frac{5 x_1}{\pi} - 6 \right)^2 + 10 \left(1 - \frac{1}{8\pi} \right) \cos(x_1) + 10$	2	$x_i \epsilon [-5, 5]$	$f(x) = 0.397887$
$f18$	Goldstein Price	$f(x) = [1 + (x_1 + x_2 + 1)^2 (19 - 14 x_1 + 3 x_1^2 - 14 x_2 + 6 x_1 x_2 + 3 x_2^2)]$ $[30 + (2 x_1 - 3 x_2)^2 (18 - 32 x_1 + 12 x_1^2 + 48 x_2 - 36 x_1 x_2 + 27 x_2^2)]$	2	$x_i \epsilon [-2, 2]$	$f(x) = 3$
$f19$	Hartmann 3D	$f(x) = -\sum\limits_{i=1}^{4} \alpha_i \exp\left(-\sum\limits_{j=1}^{3} A_{ij}(x_j - P_{ij})^2 \right)$, where $\alpha = (1.0, 1.2, 3.0, 3.2)^T$ $A = \begin{pmatrix} 3.0 & 10 & 30 \\ 0.1 & 10 & 35 \\ 3.0 & 10 & 30 \\ 0.1 & 10 & 35 \end{pmatrix}$ $P = 10^{-4} \begin{pmatrix} 3689 & 1170 & 2673 \\ 4699 & 4387 & 7470 \\ 1091 & 8732 & 5547 \\ 381 & 5743 & 8828 \end{pmatrix}$	3	$x_i \epsilon [0, 1]$	$f(x) = -3.86$
$f20$	Hartmann 6D	$f(x) = -\sum\limits_{i=1}^{4} \alpha_i \exp\left(-\sum\limits_{j=1}^{6} A_{ij}(x_j - P_{ij})^2 \right)$, where $\alpha = (1.0, 1.2, 3.0, 3.2)^T$ $A = \begin{pmatrix} 10 & 3 & 17 & 3.50 & 1.7 & 8 \\ 0.05 & 10 & 17 & 0.1 & 8 & 14 \\ 3 & 3.5 & 1.7 & 10 & 17 & 8 \\ 17 & 8 & 0.05 & 10 & 0.1 & 14 \end{pmatrix}$ $P = 10^{-4} \begin{pmatrix} 1312 & 1696 & 5569 & 124 & 8283 & 5886 \\ 2329 & 4135 & 8307 & 3736 & 1004 & 9991 \\ 2348 & 1451 & 3522 & 2883 & 3047 & 6650 \\ 4047 & 8828 & 8732 & 5743 & 1091 & 381 \end{pmatrix}$	6	$x_i \epsilon [0, 1]$	$f(x) = -3.32$
$f21$	Shekel 4.5	$f(x) = -\sum\limits_{i=1}^{5} \left(\sum\limits_{j=1}^{4} (x_j - C_{ji})^2 + \beta_i \right)^{-1}$, where $\beta = \frac{1}{10}(1, 2, 2, 4, 4, 6, 3, 7, 5, 5)^T$ $C = \begin{pmatrix} 4.0 & 1.0 & 8.0 & 6.0 & 3.0 & 2.0 & 5.0 & 8.0 & 6.0 & 7.0 \\ 4.0 & 1.0 & 8.0 & 6.0 & 7.0 & 9.0 & 5.0 & 1.0 & 2.0 & 3.6 \\ 4.0 & 1.0 & 8.0 & 6.0 & 3.0 & 2.0 & 3.0 & 8.0 & 6.0 & 7.0 \\ 4.0 & 1.0 & 8.0 & 6.0 & 7.0 & 9.0 & 3.0 & 1.0 & 2.0 & 3.6 \end{pmatrix}$	4	$x_i \epsilon [0, 10]$	$f(x) = -10.1532$
$f22$	Shekel 4.7	$f(x) = -\sum\limits_{i=1}^{7} \left(\sum\limits_{j=1}^{4} (x_j - C_{ji})^2 + \beta_i \right)^{-1}$, where $\beta = \frac{1}{10}(1, 2, 2, 4, 4, 6, 3, 7, 5, 5)^T$ $C = \begin{pmatrix} 4.0 & 1.0 & 8.0 & 6.0 & 3.0 & 2.0 & 5.0 & 8.0 & 6.0 & 7.0 \\ 4.0 & 1.0 & 8.0 & 6.0 & 7.0 & 9.0 & 5.0 & 1.0 & 2.0 & 3.6 \\ 4.0 & 1.0 & 8.0 & 6.0 & 3.0 & 2.0 & 3.0 & 8.0 & 6.0 & 7.0 \\ 4.0 & 1.0 & 8.0 & 6.0 & 7.0 & 9.0 & 3.0 & 1.0 & 2.0 & 3.6 \end{pmatrix}$	4	$x_i \epsilon [0, 10]$	$f(x) = -10.403$
$f23$	Shekel 4.10	$f(x) = -\sum\limits_{i=1}^{10} \left(\sum\limits_{j=1}^{4} (x_j - C_{ji})^2 + \beta_i \right)^{-1}$, where $\beta = \frac{1}{10}(1, 2, 2, 4, 4, 6, 3, 7, 5, 5)^T$ $C = \begin{pmatrix} 4.0 & 1.0 & 8.0 & 6.0 & 3.0 & 2.0 & 5.0 & 8.0 & 6.0 & 7.0 \\ 4.0 & 1.0 & 8.0 & 6.0 & 7.0 & 9.0 & 5.0 & 1.0 & 2.0 & 3.6 \\ 4.0 & 1.0 & 8.0 & 6.0 & 3.0 & 2.0 & 3.0 & 8.0 & 6.0 & 7.0 \\ 4.0 & 1.0 & 8.0 & 6.0 & 7.0 & 9.0 & 3.0 & 1.0 & 2.0 & 3.6 \end{pmatrix}$	4	$x_i \epsilon [0, 10]$	$f(x) = -10.5364$

Table 6. Composite benchmark functions.

f	Function	Mathematical Equation	Dimensions	Search space	Minimum
$f24$	CF1	$f_1, f_2, ..., f_{10} = Sphere\ Function$ $[\delta_1, \delta_2, ..., \delta_{10}] = [1, 1, 1, ..., 1]$ $[\lambda_1, \lambda_2, ..., \lambda_{10}] = [5/100, 5/100, ..., 5/100]$	30	$x_i \epsilon [-5, 5]$	0
$f25$	CF2	$f_1, f_2, ..., f_{10} = Griewank\ Function$ $[\delta_1, \delta_2, ..., \delta_{10}] = [1, 1, 1, ..., 1]$ $[\lambda_1, \lambda_2, ..., \lambda_{10}] = [5/100, 5/100, ..., 5/100]$	30	$x_i \epsilon [-5, 5]$	0

(*continued*)

Table 6. (*continued*)

f	Function	Mathematical Equation	Dimensions	Search space	Minimum
$f26$	CF3	$f_1, f_2, ..., f_{10} = Griewank\ Function$ $[\delta_1, \delta_2, ..., \delta_{10}] = [1, 1, 1, ..., 1]$ $[\lambda_1, \lambda_2, ..., \lambda_{10}] = [1, 1, 1, ..., 1]$	30	$x_i \epsilon\ [-5, 5]$	0
$f27$	CF4	$f_1, f_2 = Ackley\ Function$ $f_3, f_4 = Rastrigin\ Function$ $f_5, f_6 = Weierstrass\ Function$ $f_7, f_8 = Griewank\ Function$ $f_9, f_{10} = Sphere\ Function$ $[\delta_1, \delta_2, ..., \delta_{10}] = [1, 1, 1, ..., 1]$ $[\lambda_1, \lambda_2, ..., \lambda_{10}] = [5/32, 5/32, 1, 1, 5/0.5, 5/0.5, 5/100, 5/100, 5/100, 5/100]$	30	$x_i \epsilon\ [-5, 5]$	0
$f28$	CF5	$f_1, f_2 = Rastrigin\ Function$ $f_3, f_4 = Weierstrass\ Function$ $f_5, f_6 = Griewank\ Function$ $f_7, f_8 = Ackley\ Function$ $f_9, f_{10} = Sphere\ Function$ $[\delta_1, \delta_2, ..., \delta_{10}] = [1, 1, 1, ..., 1]$ $[\lambda_1, \lambda_2, ..., \lambda_{10}] = [5/32, 5/32, 1, 1, 5/0.5, 5/0.5, 5/100, 5/100, 5/100, 5/100]$	30	$x_i \epsilon\ [-5, 5]$	0
$f29$	CF6	$f_1, f_2 = Rastrigin\ Function$ $f_3, f_4 = Weierstrass\ Function$ $f_5, f_6 = Griewank\ Function$ $f_7, f_8 = Ackley\ Function$ $f_9, f_{10} = Sphere\ Function$ $[\delta_1, \delta_2, ..., \delta_{10}] = [0.1, 0.2, 0.3, 0.4, 0.5, 0.6, 0.7, 0.8, 0.9, 1]$ $[\lambda_1, \lambda_2, ..., \lambda_{10}] = [0.1 * 1/5, 0.2 * 1/5, 0.3 * 5/0.5, 0.4 * 5/0.5,$ $0.5 * 5/100, 0.6 * 5/100, 0.7 * 5/32, 0.8 * 5/32, 0.9 * 5/100, 1 * 5/100]$	30	$x_i \epsilon\ [-5, 5]$	0

4 Conclusion

In this paper, we show a multi-threaded implementation of the gray wolf algorithm. Several threads of gray wolf algorithms are executed in this new algorithm and the results are combined with four different strategies every 100 generations. The experiments with twenty-nine benchmark functions showed that our proposal was better in 17 functions and in 6 of the functions the same results were obtained as the original algorithm that is equal to the minimum reported.

Table 7. MTGWA with six threads final experiments.

Id	GWO	TB	ATB	GTB	AGTB
f1	6.590E-28	2.991E-29	6.827E-29	6.151E-29	**1.041E-28**
f2	7.180E-17	1.240E-17	2.326E-17	2.170E-17	2.665E-17
f3	3.290E-06	4.847E-27	1.033E-26	9.350E-27	1.287E-26
f4	5.610E-07	4.866E-09	9.915E-09	7.925E-09	1.176E-08
f5	26.8126	26.5574	26.4353	**26.0196**	26.2580
f6	8.1658E-01	0	0	0	0
f7	2.2130E-03	1.9221E-05	0	0	0

(*continued*)

Table 7. (*continued*)

Id	GWO	TB	ATB	GTB	AGTB
f8	−6123	−8199	−7217	−7955	**−8201**
f9	3.105E-01	8.882E-16	5.921E-17	2.961E-16	1.066E-15
f10	1.060E-13	4.296E-14	5.504E-14	3.147E-14	5.930E-14
f11	4.4850E-03	**0**	**0**	**0**	**0**
f12	5.3438E-02	2.5081E-02	2.3753E-02	1.8494E-02	2.3009E-02
f13	6.5446E-01	3.3783E-01	3.1999E-01	**2.2355E-01**	2.7501E-01
f14	4.0425	1.3948	1.2297	1.0973	1.3952
f15	3.3700E-05	3.0750E-04	3.0764E-04	3.0783E-04	3.0890E-04
f16	−1.0316	−1.0316	−1.0316	−1.0316	−1.0316
f17	0.3979	0.3979	0.3979	0.3979	0.3979
f18	3	3	3	3	3
f19	−3.8626	−3.8628	−3.8628	−3.8628	−3.8628
f20	−3.2865	−3.3224	−3.3224	−3.3224	−3.3224
f21	−10.1514	−10.1531	−10.1531	−10.1531	−10.1531
f22	−10.4015	−10.4028	−10.4028	−10.4028	−10.4028
f23	−10.5343	−10.5363	−10.5363	−10.5363	−10.5363
f24	4.384E+01	1.759E-31	4.902E-31	4.652E-31	1.277E-30
f25	9.180E+01	1.528E-15	6.200E-16	4.248E-16	4.847E-16
f26	6.144E+01	6.300E-15	2.866E-15	2.558E-15	1.598E-15
f27	123.124	432.319	335.355	483.908	559.494
f28	1.0214E+02	9.092E-17	6.666E-17	3.052E-17	5.828E-17
f29	43.143	821.745	860.151	811.769	837.791

Table 8. MTGWA with seven threads final experiments.

Id	GWO	TB	ATB	GTB	AGTB
f1	6.590E-28	1.557E-29	4.644E-29	5.045E-29	7.605E-29
f2	7.180E-17	1.135E-17	2.131E-17	1.892E-17	2.837E-17
f3	3.290E-06	3.952E-27	8.333E-27	5.157E-27	1.658E-26
f4	5.610E-07	5.252E-09	9.2246E-09	8.558E-09	1.183E-08
f5	26.8126	26.5158	26.2442	26.5281	26.1631
f6	8.1658E-01	**0**	**0**	**0**	**0**
f7	2.2130E-03	4.8910E-06	**0**	**0**	**0**
f8	−6123	−8150	−7125	−7851	−8190
f9	3.105E-01	1.184E-16	7.224E-15	**0**	2.901E-15

(continued)

Table 8. (*continued*)

Id	GWO	TB	ATB	GTB	AGTB
f10	1.060E-13	4.343E-14	4.923E-14	2.839E-14	5.267E-14
f11	4.4850E-03	**0**	**0**	**0**	**0**
f12	5.3438E-02	1.8182E-02	2.4452E-02	1.7096E-02	2.4125E-02
f13	6.5446E-01	2.8916E-01	2.9516E-01	2.3428E-01	3.6272E-01
f14	4.0425	1.1624	1.0641	1.0641	1.4285
f15	3.3700E-05	3.0749E-04	**3.0769E-04**	3.0751E-04	3.0808E-04
f16	−1.0316	−1.0316	−1.0316	−1.0316	−1.0316
f17	0.3979	0.3979	0.3979	0.3979	0.3979
f18	3	3	3	3	3
f19	−3.8626	−3.8628	−3.8628	−3.8628	−3.8628
f20	−3.2865	−3.3224	−3.3224	−3.3224	−3.3224
f21	−10.1514	−0.9832	−10.1531	−10.1531	−10.1531
f22	−10.4015	−10.4028	−10.4028	−10.4028	−10.4028
f23	−10.5343	−10.5363	−10.5363	−10.5363	−10.5363
f24	4.384E+01	**1.182E-31**	3.268E-31	4.351E-31	1.053E-30
f25	9.180E+01	1.783E-15	5.091E-16	2.509E-16	**8.106E-17**
f26	6.144E+01	6.196E-15	1.296E-15	1.550E-15	6.232E-16
f27	123.124	527.919	348.933	439.759	385.945
f28	1.0214E+02	9.29E-17	8.356E-17	2.134E-17	7.274E-17
f29	43.143	909.596	770.303	821.229	859.656

Table 9. MTGWA with eight threads final experiments.

Id	GWO	TB	ATB	GTB	AGTB
f1	6.590E-28	1.849E-29	4.920E-29	3.111E-29	7.364E-29
f2	7.180E-17	**1.085E-17**	1.833E-17	1.770E-17	2.670E-17
f3	3.290E-06	**2.215E-27**	5.244E-27	8.742E-27	1.367E-26
f4	5.610E-07	**4.316E-09**	7.917E-09	7.891E-09	9.706E-09
f5	26.8126	26.4452	26.3718	26.2147	26.1552
f6	8.1658E-01	**0**	**0**	**0**	**0**
f7	2.2130E-03	1.8666E-05	**0**	**0**	**0**
f8	−6123	−7918	−6878	−7810	−8079
f9	3.105E-01	5.921E-17	5.921E-17	3.553E-16	4.145E-16
f10	1.060E-13	4.047E-14	3.869E-14	**2.792E-14**	5.835E-14
f11	4.4850E-03	**0**	**0**	**0**	**0**

(*continued*)

Table 9. (*continued*)

Id	GWO	TB	ATB	GTB	AGTB
f12	5.3438E-02	1.8677E-02	1.9437E-02	**1.2636E-02**	1.8983E-02
f13	6.5446E-01	2.6864E-01	2.8205E-01	2.3913E-01	3.1093E-01
f14	4.0425	1.0643	1.0973	**0.9980**	1.2297
f15	3.3700E-05	3.1171E-04	3.0753E-04	3.0750E-04	3.0764E-04
f16	−1.0316	−1.0316	−1.0316	−1.0316	−1.0316
f17	0.3979	0.3979	0.3979	0.3979	0.3979
f18	3	3	3	3	3
f19	−3.8626	−3.8628	−3.8628	−3.8628	−3.8628
f20	−3.2865	−3.3224	−3.3224	−3.3224	−3.3224
f21	−10.1514	−10.1531	−10.1531	−10.1531	−10.1531
f22	−10.4015	−10.4028	−10.4028	−10.4028	−10.4028
f23	−10.5343	−10.5363	−10.5363	−10.5363	−10.5363
f24	4.384E+01	1.256E-31	3.870E-31	3.026E-31	1.013E-30
f25	9.180E+01	7.095E-16	5.730E-16	1.674E-16	8.484E-17
f26	6.144E+01	6.320E-15	9.230E-16	1.317E-15	**6.220E-16**
f27	123.124	445.452	297.489	542.278	476.529
f28	1.0214E+02	1.323E-16	6.588E-17	**1.589E-17**	5.394E-17
f29	43.143	859.377	878.409	796.441	815.896

References

1. Akhtar, S., Ahmad, A.R., Abdel-Rahman, E.M.: A metaheuristic bat-inspired algorithm for full body human pose estimation. In: 2012 9th Conference on Computer and Robot Vision, pp. 369–375 (2012)
2. Bertsimas, D., Tsitsiklis, J.: Simulated annealing. Stat. Sci. **8**, 10–15 (1993)
3. Patle, B.K., Parhi, D.R., Jagadeesh, A., Kashyap, S.K.: On firefly algorithm: optimization and application in mobile robot navigation. World J. Eng. **14**(1), 65–76 (2017). https://doi.org/10.1108/WJE-11-2016-0133
4. Dorigo, M., Blum, C.: Ant colony optimization theory: a survey. Theor. Comput. Sci. **344**(2), 243–278 (2005)
5. Eberhart, R., Kennedy, J.: A new optimizer using particle swarm theory. In: Proceedings of the 6th International Symposium on Micro Machine and Human Science, 1995. MHS 1995, pp. 39–43, October 1995
6. Henderson, D., Jacobson, S., Johnson, A.: The Theory and Practice of Simulated Annealing, pp. 287–319. Springer, Boston, April 2006. https://doi.org/10.1007/0-306-48056-5_10
7. Ingber, L.: Simulated annealing: practice versus theory. Math. Comput. Model. **18**(11), 29–57 (1993)

8. Jiang, Y., Hu, T., Huang, C., Wu, X.: An improved particle swarm optimization algorithm. Appl. Math. Comput. **193**(1), 231–239 (2007). https://doi.org/10.1016/j.amc.2007.03.047. http://www.sciencedirect.com/science/article/pii/S009630030-700392X

9. Karaboga, D., Basturk, B.: A powerful and efficient algorithm for numerical function optimization: artificial bee colony (ABC) algorithm. J. Global Optim. **39**(3), 459–471 (2007)

10. Karaboga, D., Gorkemli, B., Ozturk, C., Karaboga, N.: A comprehensive survey: artificial bee colony (ABC) algorithm and applications. Artif. Intell. Rev. **42**(1), 21–57 (2014)

11. Kirkpatrick, S., Gelatt, C.D., Vecchi, M.P.: Optimization by simulated annealing. Science **220**(4598), 671–680 (1983). https://doi.org/10.1126/science.220.4598.671. https://science.sciencemag.org/content/220/4598/671

12. Kouba, N.E.L.Y., Boudour, M.: A brief review and comparative study of nature-inspired optimization algorithms applied to power system control. In: Li, X., Wong, K.-C. (eds.) Natural Computing for Unsupervised Learning. USL, pp. 35–49. Springer, Cham (2019). https://doi.org/10.1007/978-3-319-98566-4_2

13. Koulamas, C., Antony, S., Jaen, R.: A survey of simulated annealing applications to operations research problems. Omega **22**(1), 41–56 (1994). https://doi.org/10.1016/0305-0483(94)90006-X. http://www.sciencedirect.com/science/article/pii/030504839490006X

14. Liang, J.J., Suganthan, P.N., Deb, K.: Novel composition test functions for numerical global optimization. In: Proceedings 2005 IEEE Swarm Intelligence Symposium, SIS 2005, vol. 2005, pp. 68–75, June 2005

15. Martinez-Rios, F., Murillo-Suarez, A.: A new swarm algorithm for global optimization of multimodal functions over multi-threading architecture hybridized with simulating annealing. Procedia Comput. Sci. **135**, 449–456 (2018). https://doi.org/10.1016/j.procs.2018.08.196, http://www.sciencedirect.com/science/article/pii/S1877050918314868, The 3rd International Conference on Computer Science and Computational Intelligence (ICCSCI 2018) : Empowering Smart Technology in Digital Era for a Better Life

16. Martinez-Rios, F., Murillo-Suarez, A.: Packing algorithm inspired by gravitational and electromagnetic effects. Wireless Netw. **26**(8), 5631–5644 (2019). https://doi.org/10.1007/s11276-019-02011-9

17. Memari, A., Ahmad, R., Akbari Jokar, M.R., Abdul Rahim, A.R.: A new modified firefly algorithm for optimizing a supply chain network problem. Appl. Sci. 9(1), p. 7 (2019). https://doi.org/10.3390/app9010007

18. Mirjalili, S., Mirjalili, S.M., Lewis, A.: Grey wolf optimizer. Adv. Eng. Softw. **69**, 46–61 (2014). https://doi.org/10.1016/j.advengsoft.2013.12.007. http://www.sciencedirect.com/science/article/pii/S0965997813001853

19. Mishra, S., Shaw, K., Mishra, D.: A new meta-heuristic bat inspired classification approach for microarray data. Procedia Technology **4**, 802–806 (2012). https://doi.org/10.1016/j.protcy.2012.05.131, http://www.sciencedirect.com/science/article/pii/S2212017312004100, 2nd International Conference on Computer, Communication, Control and Information Technology(C3IT-2012) on February 25 - 26, 2012

20. Muro, C., Escobedo, R., Spector, L., Coppinger, R.: Wolf-pack (canis lupus) hunting strategies emerge from simple rules in computational simulations. Behav. Process. **88**(3), 192–197 (2011). https://doi.org/10.1016/j.beproc.2011.09.006. http://www.sciencedirect.com/science/article/pii/S0376635711001884

21. Olorunda, O., Engelbrecht, A.P.: Measuring exploration/exploitation in particle swarms using swarm diversity. In: 2008 IEEE Congress on Evolutionary Computation (IEEE World Congress on Computational Intelligence), pp. 1128–1134, June 2008. https://doi.org/10.1109/CEC.2008.4630938

22. Ouyang, Z., Liu, Y., Ruan, S.J., Jiang, T.: An improved particle swarm optimization algorithm for reliability-redundancy allocation problem with mixed redundancy strategy and heterogeneous components. Reliab. Eng. Syst. Saf. **181**, 62–74 (2019). https://doi.org/10.1016/j.ress.2018.09.005. http://www.sciencedirect.com/science/article/pii/S0951832018304125

23. Rey, D., Neuhäuser, M.: Wilcoxon-signed-rank test. In: International Encyclopedia of Statistical Science, pp. 1658–1659, January 2011. https://doi.org/10.1007/978-3-642-04898-2_616

24. Socha, K., Blum, C.: An ant colony optimization algorithm for continuous optimization: application to feed-forward neural network training. Neural Comput. Appl. **16**(3), 235–247 (2007). https://doi.org/10.1007/s00521-007-0084-z

25. Tirkolaee, E.B., Alinaghian, M., Hosseinabadi, A.A.R., Sasi, M.B., Sangaiah, A.K.: An improved ant colony optimization for the multi-trip capacitated arc routing problem. Comput. Electr. Eng. **77**, 457–470 (2019). https://doi.org/10.1016/j.compeleceng.2018.01.040. http://www.sciencedirect.com/science/article/pii/S0045790617330501

26. Wang, G.G., Guo, L., Duan, H., Wang, H.: A new improved firefly algorithm for global numerical optimization. J. Comput. Theor. Nanosci. **11**, 477–485 (2014). https://doi.org/10.1166/jctn.2014.3383

27. Wang, J.S., Li, S.X.: An improved grey wolf optimizer based on differential evolution and elimination mechanism. Sci. Rep. **9**(1), 1–21 (2019). https://doi.org/10.1038/s41598-019-43546-3

28. Long, W., Xu, S.: A novel grey wolf optimizer for global optimization problems. In: 2016 IEEE Advanced Information Management, Communicates, Electronic and Automation Control Conference (IMCEC), pp. 1266–1270 (2016)

29. Yang, X.S.: A new metaheuristic bat-inspired algorithm. In: Gonzalez, J.R., Pelta, D.A., Cruz, C., Terrazas G., Krasnogor N. (eds.) Nature Inspired Cooperative Strategies for Optimization (NICSO 2010), pp. 65–74. Springer, Berlin Heidelberg (2010). https://doi.org/10.1007/978-3-642-12538-6_6

30. Yang, X.-S., He, X.: Nature-inspired optimization algorithms in engineering: overview and applications. In: Yang, X.-S. (ed.) Nature-Inspired Computation in Engineering. SCI, vol. 637, pp. 1–20. Springer, Cham (2016). https://doi.org/10.1007/978-3-319-30235-5_1

31. Zhou, J., et al.: An individual dependent multi-colony artificial bee colony algorithm. Inf. Sci. **485**, 114–140 (2019). https://doi.org/10.1016/j.ins.2019.02.014. http://www.sciencedirect.com/science/article/pii/S0020025519301239 http://www.sciencedirect.com/science/article/pii/S0020025519301239

Effectiveness of Some Tests of Spatial Randomness in the Detection of Weak Graphical Passwords in *Passpoint*

Joaquín A. Herrera-Macías[1], Lisset Suárez-Plasencia[2],
Carlos M. Legón-Pérez[3], Luis R. Piñeiro-Díaz[3], Omar Rojas[4],
and Guillermo Sosa-Gómez[4(✉)]

[1] Universidad de Matanzas, Departamento de Matemática, Matanzas, Cuba
joaquin.herrera@umcc.cu
[2] Universidad de Artemisa, Departamento de Matemática-Física, Artemisa, Cuba
l.suarez2@uart.edu.cu
[3] Universidad de la Habana, Facultad de Matemática y Computación,
Instituto de Criptografía, Habana, Cuba
clegon58@gmail.com, lrp@matcom.uh.cu
[4] Universidad Panamericana. Facultad de Ciencias Económicas y Empresariales.,
Álvaro Del Portillo 49, Zapopan, Jalisco 45010, Mexico
orojas@up.edu.mx, gsosag@up.edu.mx

Abstract. This paper explores the usability of the Ripley's K function and the nearest neighbor distance, in the detection of clustered graphical passwords in the graphical authentication stage. For it, both tests were applied to two bases of data of 10,000 clustered graphical passwords each, the first with graphical passwords clustered in an area lesser than the fourth part of the original image, the second clustered in an area lesser than eighth part of the image. The results show that none of these tests is effective in the detection of clustered graphical passwords, the reason of such failure is due to the short size of the spatial pattern in question, only the 5 points of the graphical password analyzed.

Keywords: Point pattern · Graphical password · Ripley's K function · Nearest neighbor distance · Passpoint

1 Introduction

Nowadays, graphical passwords are an important alternative to traditional alphanumeric passwords. The main reason for this is due to the fact that humans have a better ability to remember images than text [10,17]. Therefore, with graphical authentication there is no need to remember long and difficult sequences. Instead, a user can authenticate by recognizing images or parts of them. Among the graphical authentication techniques, the *Passpoint* [18,20,21] is of special interest. During the registration phase while using Passpoint, the user must select 5 points (pixels) on an image as their graphical password, each

J. A. Marmolejo-Saucedo et al. (Eds.): COMPSE 2020, LNICST 359, pp. 173–183, 2021.
https://doi.org/10.1007/978-3-030-69839-3_12

time that user wishes to authenticate they must select 5 points located in a neighborhood of the 5 points selected during registration [18,21]. The points selected as a graphical password must follow a random pattern, otherwise, they are considered weak passwords, since they can be obtained by an attacker using different techniques [6,14,17,19]. It is therefore of great importance to have a tool that warns the user during the registration phase about a possible graphical password with poor randomness.

On the other hand, we have the analysis of spatial point patterns, which is the area of spatial statistics that is dedicated to studying the characteristics of events that can be represented in a specific way in space, as well as their spatial distribution [1,8,9]. Two of the tests most used in this area to check spatial randomness are Ripley's K function test [1–3,5,8,11,13,16] and the nearest neighbor distance test [1,3,8].

Graphical passwords can be interpreted as a 5-point pattern and studied by the various techniques of the theory of spatial randomness to determine their behavior. It happens that a pattern with only 5 points seems to be a sample way too small for these techniques to work. In the literature, the smallest point pattern for which it is concluded that both tests are effective consists of 36 points [15].

In this work the effectiveness of Ripley's K function and the nearest neighbor distance technique is studied, two of the most used tests in the theory of spatial point patterns, in the scenario of graphical authentication with *Passpoint*, to validate whether or not a graphical password belongs to a random pattern. For the experiments, two databases of 10000 graphical passwords clustered on a 1920×1080 image were generated. The results obtained show that both Ripley's K function and nearest neighbor distance, are not effective tests in this scenario, due to the small sample (only 5 points); i.e., they are not able to differentiate between sets of 5 points clustered and random. All the point patterns and experiments were generated in MATLAB R2018a.

2   Preliminaries

2.1   Spatial Point Patterns

To study the distribution and behavior of phenomena that occur in specific regions of space, such as earthquakes, animal or plant populations, epidemiological information, data on human settlements, etc., its representation by means of spatial coordinates (x, y) is essential. The data set generated by these coordinates is called the *spatial pattern of points* [4,7–9,12]. From the study of the spatial pattern, the existence of interactions between the individuals of each population can be inferred.

A pattern that has special importance, in theory, is the random or Poisson pattern, which is one in which any region of the area of study has the same probability of containing a point, a definition that is equivalent to that of the distribution of Poisson. The other characteristic patterns are regular patterns, where the probability of finding a point in the vicinity of another is less than that of a random pattern; and clustered patterns, in which the probability is greater. Examples of these three traditional patterns are shown in Fig. 1.

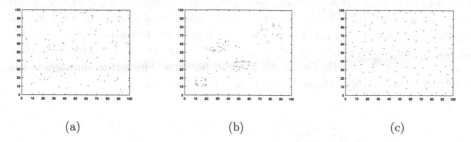

(a)   (b)   (c)

Fig. 1. Random (a), clustered (b) and regular (c) point patterns, generated in MAT-LAB.

In point pattern analysis, it is generally assumed as a null hypothesis that the pattern of points presents a random distribution, the alternative hypotheses being that the distribution might be regular [1,3,8]. Spatial point patterns have two fundamental properties: homogeneity (the pattern is translation invariant) and isotropism (the pattern is rotation invariant) [3,12]. Under these circumstances, the main characteristics of point patterns can be summarized by their first-order property, intensity: the expected number of points per unit area at any location, and by their second-order property, which describes the relationships between pairs of points.

2.2 Ripley's K Function

Ripley's K function is one of the most popular tests for spatial point pattern analysis. It is a distance-based method that measures the average number of points within a circle of radius r around any point in the pattern. It is defined as:

$$K(r) = \frac{A}{n^2} \sum_{i=1}^{n} \sum_{j=1}^{n} k_{i,j}(r) e_{i,j}(r), \quad \text{for } i \neq j,$$

where n is the number of points in the pattern, A the area of the study region, $k_{i,j}(r)$ an indicator function that takes values of 1 if the Euclidean distance between points i and j is less than r and 0 otherwise, and $e_{i,j}(r)$ is the edge correction method. Although the function $K(r)$ can be estimated without taking into account the factor $e_{i,j}(r)$, in [8] it was shown how the use of $K(r)$ without the edge correction effects lead to imprecise estimates of the pattern. However, since these methods are not perfect, it is recommended to calculate $K(r)$ for values of $r < 1/3$ of the length of the shortest side of the area of study when it has a rectangular shape [3]. A detailed review of these methods can be found in [3,8,9].

Taking into account that, in the case of regular patterns, the probability of finding a point in the vicinity of another point is lower than that of a random pattern, while in clustered patterns the probability is higher, then the interpretation of the results of $K(r)$ would be made by the comparison with the random (or Poisson) pattern πr^2 [5,8,16]. For this reason, values of $K(r) > \pi r^2$ indicate clustering, and values of $K(r) < \pi r^2$ indicate regularity, to the scale r considered. In Fig. 2 the value is represented by Ripley's K function of the three prototype patterns of Fig. 1, together with the Poisson pattern. The figure shows how the function clearly differentiates between the three patterns.

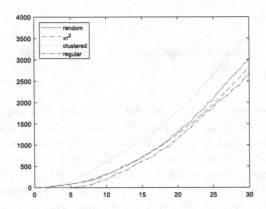

Fig. 2. Comparison of the values of Ripley's K function for the three prototypical patterns.

To facilitate the visual and numerical interpretation of the results of Ripley's K function for a given pattern, the following transformation is usually performed:

$$\hat{L}(r) = \sqrt{\frac{K(r)}{\pi}},$$

which aims to linearize the function and stabilize the variance [3,8]. Finally, the transformation $L(r) = \hat{L}(r) - r$, sets the Poisson pattern to the value 0. Consequently, a clustered pattern occurs when $L(r) > 0$ and a regular pattern occurs when $L(r) < 0$.

To perform a hypothesis test with the function $K(r)$ (or the function $L(r)$), it is necessary to estimate the critical values, we do this through Monte Carlo simulations [1,5,8,11]. We simulate a large number of random patterns with the same intensity and in the same area as the pattern under study, the value of the function is calculated for each of them and the maximum and minimum value is represented for each r reached. The null hypothesis, which would be that of complete spatial randomness (CSR), is rejected if the value of the observed function for some r falls outside the limits of the confidence interval. In some cases, it is not necessary to carry out the Monte Carlo simulation, since the critical limits of the distribution of the statistic are approximated. Ripley showed [2,3] that for $L(r)$, in rectangular study areas, the approximate critical value with a significance level of $\alpha = 0.01$ is $\pm 1.68\sqrt{A}/n$.

In Fig. 3, the function $L(r)$ is represented for each of the patterns in Fig. 1, the continuous curve represents the value of the function $L(r)$ for the pattern in question, the solid line at $L(r) = 0$ represents the theoretical value of the null hypothesis of CSR, the dashed lines represent the confidence intervals for $\alpha = 0.01$ of the test according to Ripley's approximation: $\pm 1.68\sqrt{A}/n$, the dashed lines represent the critical values obtained by 100 Monte Carlo simulations. As can be seen, for the random pattern (a), the function is within the confidence intervals, therefore the null hypothesis is accepted. For the clustered pattern (b), the function exceeds the upper limit of the confidence interval for $r > 2.5$ so the null hypothesis is rejected with a significance level of $\alpha = 0.01$ in favor of clustering for distances greater than 2.5. For the regular pattern (c), the function $L(r)$ has values less than the lower limit of the confidence interval for $r \in [2, 11]$, so the null hypothesis is also rejected in favor of grouping between the points at that scale.

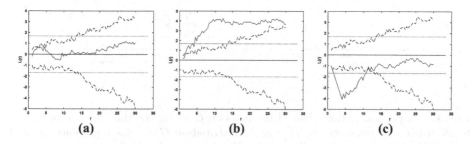

$$\text{(a)} \qquad\qquad \text{(b)} \qquad\qquad \text{(c)}$$

Fig. 3. Function $L(r)$ of the random (a), clustered (b), and regular (c) patterns of Fig. 1

2.3   Nearest Neighbor Distance

Another effective method to describe the behavior of a pattern of spatial points is the analysis of the nearest neighbor distance. If n points are randomly distributed over an area A, the expected cumulative distribution function for the nearest neighbor distances will be given by the Poisson distribution $G(d) = 1 - e^{-\lambda \pi d^2}$, where d is the distance from any point of the pattern to the closest point, and $\lambda = n/A$ its intensity. The function $G(d)$ represents the theoretical distribution of the pattern under the CSR hypothesis. To compare it with the distribution of the observed pattern, the function [1,8] is defined as

$$\hat{G}(d) = \frac{\sum_{i=1}^{n} I_i(d)}{n},$$

where n is the number of points in the pattern and $I_i(d)$ the indicator function that takes the value of 1 if the Euclidean distance between point i and its closest neighbor is less than d, and 0 otherwise.

If the point pattern is clustered, many of the distances will be small; in the same way, if it is a regular pattern, a few distances will be small. So, values of $\hat{G}(d)$ greater than the theoretical value $G(d)$ indicate clustering, while values of $\hat{G}(d)$ less than the theoretical value $G(d)$ indicate regularity [1,3,8].

As for Ripley's K function, by means of Monte Carlo simulations, the critical values of the test that allow accepting or rejecting the null hypothesis of CSR are calculated. In Fig. 4, the values of the function $\hat{G}$ are observed for each of the patterns in Fig. 1, the critical values of the test were obtained through 500 Monte Carlo simulations. The test rejects the null hypothesis for the case of the clustered and regular patterns as they are above and below the estimated critical values, respectively.

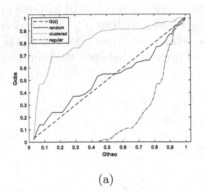 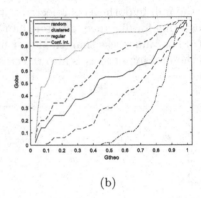

(a)   (b)

Fig. 4. Comparison of the values of the function $\hat{G}(d)$ for the three prototypical patterns, using as a reference the theoretical distribution $G(d)$ that represents the null hypothesis. It looks like the difference function between the three patterns.

3   *Passpoint* Scenario

As can be seen from the formulas of Ripley's K function and the nearest neighbor distance, their precision is directly proportional to n, but what is the minimum value of n for both tests to be considered accurate? We have not found this data in the literature consulted. In [15] both tests are applied to a 22-point pattern, the smallest pattern we have a reference for which both tests are applied; however, they did not conclude the result of said experiment or whether any of the tests were effective or not. In [15] they also experimented with a 36-point pattern for which they concluded that both tests were effective. So what will happen in the *Passpoint* scenario where patterns with only 5 points are available?

3.1   Design of the Experiment

In this work, the detection of clustering is analyzed, for which both tests were applied to two databases of clustered graphic passwords.

Database 1 (BD.1): Consists of 10000 graphical passwords generated randomly within a rectangle of 1920×1080 that satisfy that the area covered by the 5 points of each password is less than the quarter of the area of the rectangle. These passwords will be considered clustered.

Database 2 (BD.2): Also out of 10000 randomly generated graphical passwords within the 1920×1080 rectangle, each graphical password delimits an area smaller than one-eighth of the original rectangle. To discern the points BD.2 from the ones from BD.1, the aforementioned will be considered as strongly clustered.

For each of the tests, the critical values were estimated by 5000 Monte Carlo simulations of sets of 5 random points on a rectangle of size 1920×1080, in addition to Ripley's K function the confidence intervals were estimated according to Ripley's approximation $\pm 1.68\sqrt{A}/n$, where $A = 1920 * 1080$ and $n = 5$. These values for Ripley's K function can be seen in Fig. 5, the solid line at $L(r) = 0$ represents the theoretical value of the null hypothesis, the dashed lines represent the intervals of confidence for $\alpha = 0.01$ of the test according to the Ripley approximation and the dashed lines represent the critical values of the function $L(r)$ in 5000 random pattern simulations.

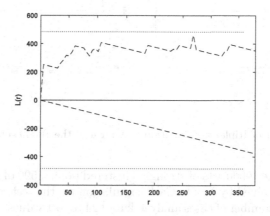

Fig. 5. Confidence intervals and critical values of Ripley's K function test for 5-point patterns.

3.2   Results

Ripley's K Test Effectiveness. Ripley's K function test applied to BD.1 shows that only 22 of the 10000 sets exceed the critical values estimated for the Monte Carlo simulation test, which represents 0.22% of all the cases analyzed, and only 1 of these sets of 5 points is above the confidence interval estimated by Ripley's approximation, which represents 0.01% of the cases analyzed. Some particular cases are shown in Fig. 6, in the first two cases it is observed how the K function is contained within the critical values, in the third, the function is above the critical values in the interval $[156, 241]$ but below the Ripley confidence interval, the fourth case is the only one in which values of the K function were obtained above the confidence interval according to Ripley's approximation for $r \in [145, 245]$.

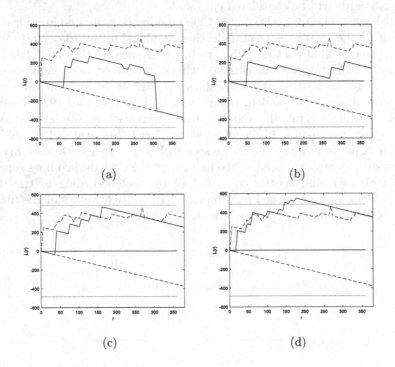

(a)   (b)

(c)   (d)

Fig. 6. Result of Ripley's K function test for 4 of the 10000 sets analyzed.

For BD.2 of the 10000 sets of strongly clustered points, 590 of them exceed the critical values obtained by Monte Carlo simulation for the test, which represents 5.9% of the total number of cases analyzed; and 24 report values of the K function greater than the confidence intervals estimated by Ripley's approximation, which represents 0.24% of the cases analyzed.

Effectiveness of the Test of the Nearest Neighbor Distance. The results obtained by the nearest neighbor distance test for BD.1 show that only 14 of the 10000 sets of 5 clustered points exceed the critical values estimated for the test by Monte Carlo simulation, which represents the 0.14% of all cases.

In the experiment with the 10000 sets of 5 strongly clustered points from BD.2, only 72 sets exceed the critical values obtained by Monte Carlo simulation, which represents 0.72% of the cases analyzed. Two particular cases are shown in the Fig. 7, in the first graph it is observed how the function $\hat{G}$ falls within the confidence intervals, therefore the CSR hypothesis is accepted; in the second, the function exceeds the value of the upper confidence interval for $d \in [16, 26]$ so the null hypothesis is rejected.

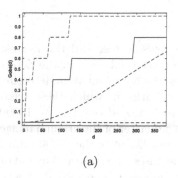

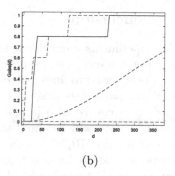

(a)   (b)

Fig. 7. Result of the nearest neighbor test for 2 of the 20000 sets analyzed.

3.3   Discussion of the Results

Both Ripley's K test and the nearest neighbor distance test were ineffective in detecting BD.1 sets as clustered. The best results were offered by Ripley's K test, which detected only 0.22% of the cases. Of these 22 sets in which the null hypothesis is rejected in the experiment, 11 of them correspond to sets of points that cover an area less than one-eighth of the image. Taking into account that, since they were not generated in a uniform way, only 194 of the 10000 sets of points of the BD.1 are in an area smaller than one-eighth of the image, then only 1.94% of cases have 50% of successes. Therefore, the function is expected to have a better success rate for the tightly clustered sets in the second database. Although these patterns of strongly clustered points are unlikely to be found in practice since it would mean selecting the 5 points in an area equivalent to one-eighth of the image area, something unlikely that a responsible user will perform, without a doubt, a graphic password with these characteristics it would offer very low security. However, experiments with BD.2 confirm the ineffectiveness of both tests in detecting clustering in 5-point patterns. Once again, the best results were obtained by Ripley's K function test, which detected 5.9% of the cases, a considerable improvement compared to the 0.22% obtained for BD.1, but still a very discreet value to be considered effective as it fails in more than 94% of the cases analyzed. These results are summarized in Table 1.

Table 1. Percentage of clustered graphical passwords detected by each test for BD.1 and BD.2

	BD.1	BD.2
Ripley's K function	0.22%	5.9%
Nearest neighbor distance	0.14%	0.72%

4   Conclusions

The experiments carried out show that both Ripley's K test and the nearest neighbor distance test, despite being some of the most used tests in the detection of clustering in finite patterns of spatial points, are not effective in detecting graphical passwords clustered in the *Passpoint* scenario, in which these passwords only consist of 5 points. The first experiment carried out for the 10000 sets of 5 points, which delimit an area smaller than a quarter of the original image area, shows that Ripley's K function test only detects 22 out of the 10000 sets of points as clustered, which represents 0.22% of the cases. The nearest neighbor distance test detected only 14 sets, for 0.14% of the cases. The second experiment, despite being with much more clustered points, since they cover an area smaller than one-eighth of the image, and yielding detection values significantly higher than those obtained for the clustered points, also shows the inefficiency of both tests in the *Passpoint* scenario since of the 10000 strongly clustered sets simulated Ripley's K function test only detects 590, which represents 5.9% of the cases; while the closest neighbor detected 72, for 0.72% of the cases.

Since these two spatial pattern analysis techniques are not effective in detecting clustering in the graphical authentication scenario with *Passpoint*, it is necessary to develop methods to detect clustering in graphical passwords of only 5 points, which it would allow users to warn about a possible weak graphical password. The use of some of the improved variants of these tests could be explored, but taking into account the small sample size, our future research will be directed in another direction, the development of new methods that allow detecting clustering in the said scenario with high reliability.

References

1. Caballero Pérez, Y.B.: Test de aleatoriedad para procesos puntuales espaciales basado en el cálculo de la dimensión fractal. Estadística (2017)
2. Casanova, M.R., Orts, V., Albert, J.M., Mateu, J.: Distance-based methods: Ripley's k function vs. k density function. Tech. rep., European Regional Science Association (2011)
3. De La Cruz, M.: Métodos para analizar datos puntuales. Introd. al Análisis Espac. Datos en Ecol. y Ciencias Ambient. Métodos y Apl., pp. 75–127 (2008). https://dialnet.unirioja.es/servlet/articulo?codigo=2771482
4. Diggle, P.J.: Statistical Analysis of Spatial and Spatio-temporal Point Patterns. 3rd edition. CRC Press (2013). https://doi.org/10.1201/b15326
5. Dixon, P.M.: Ripley's K function. In: Wiley StatsRef Stat. Ref. Online. John Wiley & Sons, Ltd. (2014). https://doi.org/10.1002/9781118445112.stat07751
6. Gao, H., Jia, W., Ye, F., Ma, L.: A survey on the use of graphical passwords in security. J. Softw. **8**(7), 1678–1698 (2013). https://doi.org/10.4304/jsw.8.7.1678-1698
7. Gelfand, A., Diggle, P., Guttorp, P., Fuentes, M.: Handbook of spatial statistics. Handb. Spat. Stat. (2010). https://doi.org/10.1201/9781420072884
8. Gómez-Rubio, V.: Spatial Point Patterns: Methodology and Applications with R. J. Stat. Softw. 75(Book Review 2) (2016). https://doi.org/10.18637/jss.v075.b02, http://www.spatstat.org/

9. Illian, J., Penttinen, A., Stoyan, H., Stoyan, D.: Statistical Analysis and Modelling of Spatial Point Patterns. vol. 70. John Wiley & Sons (2008). https://doi.org/10. 1002/9780470725160

10. Itti, L., Koch, C.: Computational modelling of visual attention. Nat. Rev. Neurosci. **2**(3), 194–203 (2001). https://doi.org/10.1038/35058500, https://www. nature.com/articles/35058500

11. Kopczewska, K.: Cluster-based measurement of agglomeration, concentration and specialisation. Measuring Regional Specialisation, pp. 69–171. Springer, Cham (2017). https://doi.org/10.1007/978-3-319-51505-2_2

12. Nakoinz, O., Knitter, D.: Modelling Human Behaviour in Landscapes. QAAM. Springer, Cham (2016). https://doi.org/10.1007/978-3-319-29538-1

13. Ripley, B.D.: Tests of 'Randomness' for spatial point patterns. J. R. Stat. Soc. Ser. B **41**(3), 368–374 (1979). https://doi.org/10.1111/j.2517-6161.1979.tb01091.x

14. Rittenhouse, R.G., Chaudry, J.A., Lee, M.: Security in graphical authentication. Int. J. Secur. Its Appl. **7**(3), 347–356 (2013)

15. Rozas, V., Camarero, J.: Técnicas de análisis espacial de patrones de puntos aplicadas en ecología forestal. Forest Syst. **14**(1), 79–97 (2008)

16. Schabenberger, O., Gotway, C.A.: Statistical Methods for Spatial Data Analysis. CRC Press (2017). https://doi.org/10.1201/9781315275086

17. Valdés, O.R., Legón, C.C.M., Socorro, C.R., Navarro, P.: Patrones en el orden de los clics y su influencia en la debilidad de las claves en la Técnica de Autenticacion Gráfica Passpoints. IV Semin. Cient\ifico Nac. Criptograf\ia (2018)

18. Valdés, O.R., Legón, C.M., Llanes, R.S.: Seguridad y usabilidad de los esquemas y técnicas de autenticación gráfica. Rev. Cubana Cien. Inform. **12**, 13–27 (2018)

19. Van Oorschot, P.C., Thorpe, J.: Exploiting predictability in click-based graphical passwords. J. Comput. Secur. **19**(4), 699–702 (2011). https://doi.org/10.3233/ JCS-2010-0411

20. Wiedenbeck, S., Waters, J., Birget, J.C., Brodskiy, A., Memon, N.: Authentication using graphical passwords: effects of tolerance and image choice. ACM Int. Conf. Proc. Ser. **93**, 1–12 (2005). https://doi.org/10.1145/1073001.1073002

21. Wiedenbeck, S., Waters, J., Birget, J.C., Brodskiy, A., Memon, N.: PassPoints: design and longitudinal evaluation of a graphical password system. Int. J. Hum. Comput. Stud. **63**(1–2), 102–127 (2005). https://doi.org/10.1016/j.ijhcs.2005.04. 010

Analysis of the Number of Sides of Voronoi Polygons in PassPoint

Lisset Suárez-Plasencia[1], Joaquín A. Herrera-Macías[2],
Carlos M. Legón-Pérez[3], Raisa Socorro-LLanes[4], Omar Rojas[5],
and Guillermo Sosa-Gómez[5(✉)]

[1] Departamento de Matemática-Física, Universidad de Artemisa, Artemisa, Cuba
l.suarez2@uart.edu.cu
[2] Departamento de Matemática, Universidad de Matanzas, Matanzas, Cuba
joaquin.herrera@umcc.cu
[3] Facultad de Matemática y Computación, Instituto de Criptografía,
Universidad de la Habana, Habana, Cuba
clegon58@gmail.com
[4] Facultad de Informática, Universidad Tecnológica de la Habana, Habana, Cuba
raisa@ceis.cujae.edu.cu
[5] Facultad de Ciencias Económicas y Empresariales, Universidad Panamericana,
Álvaro del Portillo 49, 45010 Zapopan, Jalisco, Mexico
{orojas,gsosag}@up.edu.mx

Abstract. The probabilistic distribution of the characteristics of
Voronoi polygons has been extensively studied due to its many areas of
application. In various works that differ in the number of polygons generated and in the size of their regions, it is concluded that the expected
value of the characteristic number of sides of Voronoi polygons is equal
to 6. In this work, this characteristic in the polygons generated by the
graphical passwords of the graphical authentication system *PassPoint* is
studied. Its distribution is estimated and it is shown that the expected
value of the number of sides of the Voronoi polygons in this scenario
differs from previous works. The effectiveness of this feature is evaluated
to detect weak graphical passwords made up of grouped dots. They are
to be detected by estimating the entropy of the number of sides and by
the expected value of the number of sides. It is concluded that the distribution of the number of sides in this scenario does not the 3-parameter
gamma distribution reported in previous work or any of 61 distributions that were tested, and that the entropy and the expected value of
the number of sides are not efficient for the detection of weak graphical
passwords of *PassPoint* formed by 5 grouped points.

Keywords: Passpoint · Voronoi polygons · Entropy

1 Introduction

The antecedents of the Voronoi diagrams date back to the 17th century, when
the French mathematician Rene Descartes, in his work *Principia Philosophiae*

© ICST Institute for Computer Sciences, Social Informatics and Telecommunications Engineering 2021
Published by Springer Nature Switzerland AG 2021. All Rights Reserved
J. A. Marmolejo-Saucedo et al. (Eds.): COMPSE 2020, LNICST 359, pp. 184–200, 2021.
https://doi.org/10.1007/978-3-030-69839-3_13

published in 1644, describes a partition of the universe's discs into 'vortices'. Although he does not explicitly define his vortexes in the manner of Voronoi cells (regions), his work is conceptually very similar [2,36]. The first references on the subject were known in 2003, because his idea did not coincide with that of the mathematicians of that time. In the 19th century, the Voronoi diagram was conceptually formalized by the German mathematician Johann Peter Gustav Lejeune Dirichlet for the 2D and 3D cases, and extended at the beginning of the next century by the Russian mathematician Georges Voronoi for the n-dimensional case [36]. These diagrams are nothing more than a geometric structure studied in computational geometry, which represents approximate information about a set of points called sites or generators. Voronoi (or Thiessen) diagrams or polygons (as they are also often called) are known in different ways due to their immense applications in various branches of science, including computation, meteorology, physics, geology, crystallography, anthropology, among others [2,36]. Recently, in [26] and [39] they have been used in graphical authentication and robotics respectively.

The dual of a 2D Voronoi diagram is a Delaunay triangulation (or Delaunay mosaic), and was exposed before 1872 by the French mathematician Charles Delaunay [36]. These diagrams and their dual, present a set of characteristics determined by the properties of randomness or dependence of the initial set of points. Polygons where their points follow a random distribution are called *Voronoi Poisson polygons* [8–11,16,17,20].

One of the main applications of Voronoi polygons using their characteristics is to evaluate randomness or detect the existence of patterns in the initial set of points [37]. According to on the behavior of the points distributed in the plane, the spatial point patterns are classified as random (homogeneous Poisson point process), regular (uniform or an inhibiting pattern) or grouped (aggregated), see [3,11,18,32,37,47].

In [11], a set of these characteristics was investigated for the existence of patterns, however the exclusion of the number of sides of the Voronoi polygons from the set of investigated characteristics is not argued. On the other hand, in [22] it was shown that the K-Ripley function and the distance to the nearest neighbor, two of the most used tests in spatial randomness, are inefficient to detect clustering in graphical passwords in the system *PassPoint* (which is based on the user remembering 5 dot patterns on an image selected as their password) [29,41,48]. In this system, a password is considered weak if the 5 points selected by the user do not follow a random distribution. The main types of non-randomness that may be present between the points in that case are: grouping, regularity, smoothness, and symmetry. By the results of [11] and [22] the efficiency of the characteristic number of sides of Voronoi polygons, to detect graphical passwords with points grouped in *PassPoint* is investigated in this work.

The numerous applications of the Voronoi polygons in different areas of knowledge have generated a great variety of studies on their characteristics and their proballistic distribution. These distributions, as well as those of the characteristics of the Delaunay triangulations in the two-dimensional case, are unknown in many cases, and it is necessary to apply simulation techniques to estimate them [7,8,11,13,14,23,24,28,38,46].

In [10,20,21], some theoretical results associated with the distribution of the number of sides of the Voronoi polygons. In [7,8,11,13,14,23,24,28,46] the distribution of the number of sides of the Voronoi Poisson polygons is estimated by simulation. Despite being generated in these studies between 200 and 208,969,210 of Voronoi Poisson polygons in a given region of the plane, the expected value does not vary, it is always 6 [7,8,11,13,14,23,24,28,46]. In [6], to measure the level of uniformity of the obtained polygons, the probability P_N is defined as the proportion of polygons with N sides and to this distribution $\{P_N | \Sigma_N P_N = 1\}$ of the number of sides, the Voronoi entropy $S_{vor} = H(P_N) = -\Sigma P_N \log P_N$ is calculated, which allows quantify the ordering of the set of points in the plane or the cells around these points.

On the other hand, in graphical authentication, entropy is used as a measure of complexity, the amount of information in an image, or the security of a password. This is especially useful when estimating whether an image is useful for the authentication process using the *PassPoint* system. In [27], it is concluded that image passwords with high entropy are easy to forget, or what is the same difficult to remember the password.

In this work a state of the art distribution of the characteristics of Voronoi polygons is presented, in particular on the characteristic number of sides. It is investigated, for the first time as far as we know, in a very peculiar scenario: the polygons generated by the graphical passwords used in the *PassPoint* graphical authentication system, where it is only possible to generate 5 polygons on a rectangular area of the flat. The distribution of this characteristic in this scenario is estimated and its effectiveness in detecting weak graphical passwords formed by grouped points is evaluated.

The work is structured in 6 sections: Section 1 shows the Introduction; Section 2 is composed by Voronoi polygons and *PassPoint*; Section 3 shows the background of the distribution of some characteristics of the Voronoi polygons and specifically the background of the distribution of the number of sides of the Voronoi Poisson polygons; Section 4 presents our main contribution: Analysis of the number of sides of Voronoi polygons in *PassPoint*; Section 5 show the comparison with previous works; and finally in Section 6 the conclusions are presented.

2   Preliminaries

2.1   Voronoi Polygons

Voronoi diagrams are a geometric construct that, given a set $P = \{p_1, p_2, \ldots, p_n\}$ of n points, called sites, allows to build a partition of the Euclidean plane in a set of n disjoint regions, so that each region $V(p_i)$ corresponds to a single site p_i. The points q belonging to a given region $V(p_i)$ fulfill the property of being at a lower (Euclidean) distance from the site p_i corresponding to that region than to any other site p_j; i.e., $d(q, p_i) \leq d(q, p_j)$, $\forall p_i \neq p_j, 1 \leq i, j \leq n$. In Voronoi diagrams not all regions are bounded, the bounded ones are known as closed Voronoi polygons (V.P.) or convex polygons, and the unbounded ones as unbounded regions or open Voronoi polygons. The boundaries of the Voronoi regions are defined by bisectors joining each pair of sites, and the point of intersection between the bisectors is called the Voronoi vertex. In [5,15,19,30,38,45], the Voronoi regions are also often referred to as Voronoi cells, the boundaries as edges, the sites by generating points, and the set formed by these points is called the generator set.

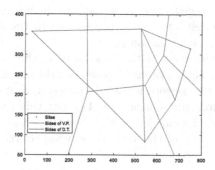

Fig. 1. Representation of a Voronoi diagram and its dual.

The dual of a two-dimensional Voronoi diagram is a Delaunay triangulation (D.T.), see Fig. 1. This triangulation is performed by connecting to the closest vertices, satisfying that all circumscribed circles in the network of triangles are empty, this restriction is known as the Delaunay condition. If P is a randomly generated set of the plane, then the Voronoi polygons and Delaunay triangulations are random, called Voronoi polygons and Delaunay Poisson triangulations [7,8,11,13,14,23,24,28,38,46].

Voronoi polygons and their Delaunay triangulations have a set of characteristics determined by the properties of randomness or dependence on the initial set of points. In the two-dimensional case, these characteristics are the following [11,38]:

- N number of sides (edges or vertices) of the polygons
- Length L_V of a side of a Voronoi polygon
- Length L_D of a side of a Delaunay triangle
- Distance R between a site and a vertex of its Voronoi polygon (R radius of a circle circumscribed in a Delaunay triangle)
- Area A_D and perimeter P_D of a Delaunay triangle
- Area A_V and perimeter P_V of a Voronoi polygon
- Interior angle α_{int} of a Delaunay triangle
- Minimum angle α_{min}, mean angle α_{med} and maximum angle α_{max} of a Delaunay triangle

In [11] the characteristics were analyzed, α_{max}, α_{med}, α_{int}, L_V, R, A_D, P_D, L_D and α_{min}, given an initial set of 100 clustered or regular patterns in a square unit, concluding that the first eight characteristics are more competent to detect clustering and the last regularity [11].

2.2 PassPoint

The *PassPoint* [29,41,48] system is one of the most advantageous techniques of the *cued-recall* type in graphical authentication, due to its security and usability. This technique requires the user to select an ordered set of 5 pixels in an image as their password in the registration phase, and in the authentication phase they must select "approximately" the same pixels, and in the same order in which they were selected in the registration phase.

In graphical authentication with *PassPoint*, if the set of points (pixels) selected by the user as their graphical password do not follow a random pattern, then said graphical password is considered weak, as it can be compromised by so-called attacks from dictionaries [40,41]. For this reason, it is necessary to detect user selection of weak passwords. For this reason, it would be useful to evaluate the effectiveness of the Voronoi polygon characteristics in detecting patterns in *PassPoint*.

3 Background of the Distribution of Some Characteristics of the Voronoi Polygons

For many features of Voronoi polygons and Delaunay Poisson triangulations, their distributions are unknown and have been approximated by simulation, but in some cases theoretical results are already known. In [16] and [35], they report the estimated probability density functions for the minimum angle α_{min} and the edge length L_D of a Delaunay Poisson triangle with intensity $\lambda = \dfrac{N(A)}{|A|}$, ($N(A)$ number of points distributed in the study area A) [18] respectively. In [23] and [46], they obtained the first four moments of N, A_V, P_V and α_{int} from a Voronoi polygon and later adapted their histograms to a Gamma generalized three-parameter distribution; to estimate the parameters of the generalized Gamma distribution of three parameters in [46] they used the maximum likelihood estimator. A summary of various previous works, before the year 2000, on the study of some of the characteristics of Voronoi Poisson polygons by simulation is found in Table 5.4.1 of [38]. For the number of sides, Hayen and Quine in [20,21] presented an integral formula for $\hat{p}_3$ (probability associated with the number of side 3), obtaining in [20] a value of 7 decimal places and soon in [21] the improved value for 10 decimal places, $\hat{p}_3 = 0.0112400129$. In 2002, Calka [10] using a technique based on the famous formula given by Slivnyak in [34], proved an explicit expression (an integral formula) for the distribution function of the number of sides of a polygon of Voronoi Poisson, where the value of $\hat{p}_3$ in [20,21] matches the value of [10].

3.1   Background of the Distribution of the Number of Sides of the Voronoi Poisson Polygons

In previous works that estimate the distribution of the number of sides of Voronoi Poisson polygons through simulation, two fundamental variants of estimating the number of sides of Voronoi polygons are observed:

- The first variant consists of the simulation of n polygons in n iterations, generating in each of the iterations a set of m random points in a given rectangular region, in which only the number of sides of the polygon is extracted Voronoi associated to the point closest to the center of the region to avoid the edge effect.
- In the second variant, n polygons are generated in a set of the plane, with n relatively "big" neglecting the polygons that are partially bounded by an edge of the study area, calling said edge cause effect [33].

Despite their different estimation methods, their probabilities roughly correspond to the theoretical distribution of the number of sides of the Voronoi polygons found in [10].

Variant 1. In [14], Crain generated a total of 46,000 Voronoi Poisson polygons, to which he added the results of the generation of 11,000 polygons that he had previously published in [13], conducting a study of the number of sides of the 57,000 Voronoi Poisson polygons associated with the points closest to the center. For the simulation of these polygons, he generated a set of 35 random points in a square unit because it was the maximum number of points that could be generated when compiling. Hinde and Miles in [23], to estimate with better precision the properties of the distribution of the number of sides, simulated in n iterations, 2,000,000 Voronoi Poisson polygons associated to the points closest to the center of the rectangle, in each one of them they generated over a rectangular region of the plane Voronoi polygons with intensity $\lambda = 100$. In [24], they simulated 100 Voronoi Poisson polygons in a square of dimensions 25×25, with units of arbitrary length and intensity $\lambda = 0.16$. To do this, they subdivided the initial square into squares of 5×5, and in each one they generated 4 sites such that the minimum distance to any other site of the square of 25×25 was greater than a set value, in the case of random points they established the parameter from $\delta = 0.0$ up to $\delta = 0.1$. Kumar and Kurtz [28] reported a simulation of 650,000 Voronoi Poisson polygons in 650,000 iterations, for this they defined a square region in which they generated 100 random points with one of the points in the center of the square, then they calculated the properties of the Voronoi polygons associated with the center point. Tanemura [46] performed basically the same procedure as Hinde and Miles [23], but unlike them, he generated 10,000,000 Voronoi Poisson polygons, for an intensity $\lambda = 200$, in a given region of the plane simulated a number of Voronoi Poisson polygons by estimating only the number of sides of the polygons corresponding to the center point.

Variant 2. In [8], the antecedent with the highest number of simulated polygons is reported, Brakke reports a simulation of 208,969,210 Voronoi Poisson polygons in the plane. In a square unit he generated 88 polygons per second, for a total of approximately 3,801,600 polygons per day, simulating the number of polygons estimated in 55 days. Schmid and Leitner in [44], simulated 100,000 in 100,000 Voronoi Poisson polygons in a rectangular area of approximately 33 × 17, sampling up to 1,000,000 Voronoi polygons. To estimate the number of sides of the observed Voronoi polygons, the edges of the study area were not taken into account, the open polygons being discarded by the edge effect. In [7], Bormashenko, Legchenkova, and Frenkel generated a set of 200 random points in a circle of a given diameter, obtaining a Voronoi entropy equal to 1.65.

The studies carried out in [7,8] and [44] of the number of sides of the Voronoi Poisson polygons, unlike the rest of the antecedents, generate in the same iteration a relatively "large quantity" of polygons. However, their probabilities correspond approximately to the previous ones and the expected value associated with this characteristic is always 6, (see Table 1).

Table 1. Distribution and expected value of the number of sides the Voronoi polygons of the antecedents, except those obtained in [7,44] because they do not explicitly give their exact values, and those of [24] are not known.

N	$\hat{p}_N$ (Crain, 1978)	$\hat{p}_N$ (Hinde & Miles, 1980)	$\hat{p}_N$ (Kumar & Kurtz, 1993)	$\hat{p}_N$ (Calka, 2002)	$\hat{p}_N$ (Tanemura, 2003)	$\hat{p}_N$ (Brakke, 2005)
3	0.011000	0.01131	0.01100	0.011240	0.01125	0.01125
4	0.107800	0.10710	0.10710	0.106838	0.10685	0.10683
5	0.259400	0.25910	0.26000	0.259460	0.25941	0.25945
6	0.295200	0.29440	0.29400	0.294730	0.29479	0.29471
7	0.198400	0.19910	0.19900	0.198770	0.19884	0.19880
8	0.089600	0.09020	0.09000	0.089700	0.09003	0.09012
9	0.029600	0.02950	0.03000	0.029500	0.02963	0.02964
10	0.007510	0.00743	0.00700	0.000000	0.00743	0.00745
11	0.001420	0.00149	0.00150	0.000000	0.00149	0.00148
12	0.000175	0.00025	0.00023	0.000000	0.00025	0.00024
13	0.000053	0.00003	0.00004	0.000000	0.00003	0.00003
$E[N]$	6	6	6	6	6	6

Regarding its distribution, as early as in 1980, Hinde and Miles shown that the distribution of the number of sides adjusts to a generalized three parameter Gamma (3P) distribution. Later, in 2003, Tanemura [46] estimated the parameters of said distribution, where $\hat{a} = 0.96853$, $\hat{b} = 3.80078$ and $\hat{c} = 20.86016$.

4   Analysis of the Number of Sides of Voronoi Polygons in *PassPoint*

In the aforementioned previous works, the different scenarios of each study are reflected to estimate the number of sides of the Voronoi polygons, avoiding the edge effect [33] in each one. In [25] they analyzed the relationship between the proportion of points that must be excluded and the number of points in a given area using Monte-Carlo simulation, turning out to be very few points not excluded if the number of points is less than 25.

4.1   Differences of the Polygons of This Scenario with Previous Studies

In this work, the study area will be rectangular images, which can only be partitioned into 5 polygons, corresponding to the 5 points of the password of *PassPoint*. For this reason, at least 4 of these Voronoi polygons can remain open, but if the open polygons are neglected to avoid the edge effect, only one polygon at most should remain, and if the number of sides of the closest Voronoi polygons were estimated, the center would be the risk of being an open polygon. Therefore, the edges of the images will be taken into account when estimating the number of sides to obtain closed Voronoi polygons.

4.2   Design of the Experiment

The analyzes are performed for two image sizes, 800×480 and 1366×768 pixels, as they are the most common on mobile phones and computers, respectively. For each image, two databases of 300 random graphic passwords (R.G.P.) each were generated in *PassPoint*, with intensity $\lambda = 1.3021 \times 10^{-5}$ and $\lambda = 4.7660 \times 10^{-6}$, respectively, for a total of 1,500 closed Voronoi-Poisson polygons in each case. The estimation of the distribution of the number of sides of the Voronoi polygons was done without taking into account the order in which the pixels are selected by the user. The experiments carried out were developed in the R2018a version of Matlab. For each password in each database, the image was divided into the 5 Voronoi polygons, corresponding to the password points, and the number of sides, N, of each of the 1,500 polygons obtained in the 300 passwords of the 5 points each. The results are shown below.

4.3   Expected Value of the Number of Sides of the Voronoi Polygons in the Graphical Passwords of *PassPoint*

By partitioning the selected images into Voronoi polygons, with their corresponding random database, and counting the number of sides N of the Voronoi polygons associated with each of the pixels in the password, Table 2 is presented. The first database (DB.1) belongs to the image with size 800×480 pixels and to the second database (DB.2) the most frequent dimension in computers. These table is organized by the numbers of sides from highest to lowest absolute frequency to show the numbers of sides that are more (4 and 5), less (6 and 3) and not (7) significant, which can be observed in Fig. 2. Using said table and figure, it is also possible to perceive the fit between the estimated distributions, due to the overlap between both databases provided by the accumulated frequency and the Fig. 2.

Table 2. Observed frequencies of the occurrence of the number of sides in the DB. 1 and 2 respectively.

N	Frequencies DB.1	Frequencies DB.2	Relative F.(R.F.) DB.2	1-Cum.R.F DB.2
4	648	660	0.44000	0.56000
5	595	605	0.40333	0.15667
6	148	131	0.08733	0.06934
3	100	96	0.06400	0.00534
7	9	8	0.00534	0.00000
Total	1500	1500	1	–

The expected values and the variances associated with the random variable (number of sides) for DB.1 and DB.2 are, $E[N] = 4.5453$ and $E[N] = 4.53$, and $V[N] = 0.6147$ and $V[N] = 0.5838$ respectively. Note that both expected values are approximately 4.5 and the variances approximately 0.6 despite the differences between the intensities.

4.4   Evaluation of the Effectiveness of the Number of Sides of the Voronoi Polygons to Detect Clustering in the Graphical Passwords of *PassPoint*

In this subsection, a test based on the number of sides of the Voronoi polygons is proposed to detect grouping of points in the graphical passwords of *PassPoint*.

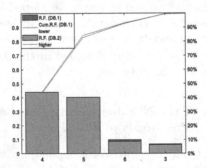

Fig. 2. Pareto diagram of the most and least significant numbers of sides observed in DB.1 and DB.2 respectively.

4.4.1 Proposal of a Randomness Test Based on the Number of Sides of the Voronoi Polygons in *PassPoint*

The following hypotheses are proposed: H_0: The password points have been selected at random and H_1: Otherwise, with test statistic given by the number of sides of the Voronoi polygons generated by the password selected by the user. The critical region defined from the numbers of sides that appear less frequently in graphical passwords whose points are random. There are 3 possible options: CR.1: $\{N > 6\}$, CR.2: $\{N = 3\} \cup \{N > 6\}$, CR.3: $\{N = 3\} \cup \{N > 5\}$.

4.4.2 Evaluation of the Effectiveness of the Test

To evaluate the effectiveness of the proposed test, type I and type II errors were measured.

Table 3. Probability estimated in DB.2.1, that the side number belongs to the critical region $(CR.)$ under the hypothesis of randomness.

Acceptance region	H_0 rejection region $(CR.)$	$\hat{p}(N \in CR. \mid H_0)$ DB.2.1
$3 \leq N \leq 6$	$\{N > 6\}$	0.00667
$4 \leq N \leq 6$	$\{N = 3\} \cup \{N > 6\}$	0.07934
$4 \leq N \leq 5$	$\{N = 3\} \cup \{N > 5\}$	0.18267

In Table 3, due to the adjustment of the distribution of the number of sides between DB.1 and DB.2, only a new database (DB.2.1) of 300 random graphical passwords was generated in an image with a size of 1366×768 pixels to estimate the type I error.

Note that since each graphical password is made up of 5 Voronoi polygons, it may be the case that a graphical password contains 0, 1, or more than 2 or more polygons whose number of sides belongs to the reject region.

As for the decision criteria, the graphical password selected by the user does not follow a random pattern if in the Voronoi polygons generated by it, there is at least a polygon with the number of sides that belongs to the rejection region. The graphical password follows a random pattern if all the side numbers of the Voronoi polygons generated do not belong to the rejection region, or they all belong to the acceptance region.

A new database (DB.3) of 300 grouped graphical passwords (G.G.P.) was generated in one sixteenth of the image of size 1366×768 pixels, and the proposed test was applied to each of the passwords, results shown in Table 4.

As can be seen in Table 4, for each of the 3 rejection regions, the proportion of passwords with grouped points that are rejected by the proposed test is very small. The highest effectiveness is obtained for CR.3, with a 53% rejection, which is still insufficient.

Table 4. Number of rejected graphical passwords (G.G.P.) observed in DB.3.

Rejection region of H_0	Number and proportion of G.G.P. detected in DB. 3
$\{N > 6\}$	8/300 = 0.0266
$\{N = 3\} \cup \{N > 6\}$	85/300 = 0.2833
$\{N = 3\} \cup \{N > 5\}$	159/300 = 0.5300

Comparison of the Histograms of the Number of Sides for DB.2 and DB.3

The low effectiveness of the proposed test is also explained by the overlap of both distributions (by means of the green) illustrated in the following graph (Fig. 3).

4.5   Distribution and Evaluation of the Entropy of the Number of Sides of the Voronoi Polygons in the Graphical Passwords of *PassPoint*

In this subsection the fit between the estimated probabilities of the number of sides of the Voronoi polygons is measured for the random databases (Table 2) and the 54 theoretical distributions which supports the EasyFit 5.6 program [42, 43], with some of them for various parameter sets for a total of 61 distributions. This program allows you to automatically fit the distributions to the sample data and select the best model in a few seconds.

For the distribution of the number of sides of the polygons of the graphical passwords formed by 5 random points and contained in DB.1 and DB.2, sets of parameters other than those of Tanemura are obtained in [46] for a generalized gamma function of 3P, $\hat{\alpha}_1 = 55.219$, $\hat{\beta}_1 = 0.10566$, $\hat{\gamma}_1 = -1.2878$ and $\hat{\alpha}_2 = 59.359$, $\hat{\beta}_2 = 0.09934$, $\hat{\gamma}_2 = -1.3664$, respectively. When the Kolmogorov-Smirnov, Anderson-Darling and χ^2 tests are performed, they are rejected with

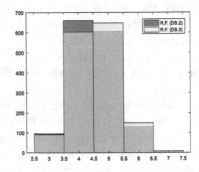

Fig. 3. Histograms of the observed frequencies of the number of sides of the Voronoi polygons in the random (DB.2) and clustered (DB.3) graphical passwords. (Color figure online)

significance levels $\alpha = \{0.2, 0.1, 0.05, 0.02, 0.01\}$ and a $p - value = 0$. The test statistics obtained for DB.1 were 0.24819, 103.22 and 720.95, respectively, and those of DB.2, 0.25289, 108.88 and 710.42, respectively. This result differs from those obtained in [23] and [46]. Even these distributions did not fit any of the 60 remaining distributions that this software brings by default.

4.5.1   Estimation of Entropy

In graphical authentication, entropy is used to measure the security of the password. In [4,29] they use the formula for the calculation: $H(x) = Nlog_2(\| L \| O \| C \|)$, where N is the number of runs, L the Locus alphabet, O the target alphabet and C the alphabet color. For this they assume equiprobable passwords and maximum entropy and illustrate in [4] a comparison between some graphical authentication systems, including the *Passpoint*. But, dictionary attacks on these systems do not traverse the equally likely (randomly distributed) passwords, as they restrict their search space by selecting the most probable passwords. Therefore, their approach does not measure resistance against dictionary attacks with non-equiprobable password traversing.

To measure the level of uncertainty of this characteristic in random and grouped graphical passwords in *PassPoint*, the entropy will depend on the probabilities of the estimated number of sides. The entropy of said characteristic was estimated using parametric, non-parametric and semi-parametric estimators. A description and comparison of these estimators can be seen in [12]. In the background, when they calculate the entropy associated with the number of sides they only use the maximum likelihood estimator (ML) [6,7,31], although it is known to be a biased estimator. Also in [6,7] they call it Voronoi entropy, but this name is not correct because the entropy they used to measure the information is known as Shannon entropy. In this work, other estimators are used for a better estimation, the parametrics calculated were the Bayesian estimators Jeffreys, Laplace, Schürman-Grassberger, Minimax and finally the semi-parametric Shrink estimator [1].

To find the entropy estimators in a sample of 300 graphical, random and grouped passwords, these estimators were calculated for each of the passwords in the size image, 1366×768 pixels. The 5 different probability distributions associated with the side numbers that appear in the 300 passwords for the two databases coincide, and therefore their entropies. Although only the probability distributions shown in the Table 5 appeared, this does not mean that the following probabilities [0; 1; 0; 0; 0] and [1/5; 1/5; 1/5; 1/5; 1/5] might not be possible.

Table 5. Frequencies of appearance $(F.A)$ of the distributions in each type of database (random (DB.2) and clustered (DB.3)) and the entropy estimators (calculated in bits) associated with the number of sides of the 300 graphical passwords in each DB.

$\hat{p}_N$	F.(R.G.P)	F.(G.G.P)	$\hat{H}^{ML}$	$\hat{H}^{Bayes}_{JEF}$	$\hat{H}^{Bayes}_{LAP}$	$\hat{H}^{Bayes}_{SG}$	$\hat{H}^{Bayes}_{Minimax}$	$\hat{H}^{Bayes}_{Shrink}$
$[1/5; 4/5; 0; 0; 0]$	0.1033	0.0767	0.7219	1.6879	1.9610	1.3153	1.6407	1.1409
$[2/5; 3/5; 0; 0; 0]$	0.4533	0.4300	0.9710	1.8228	2.0464	1.5051	1.7832	1.3521
$[2/5; 2/5; 1/5; 0; 0]$	0.1100	0.0933	1.5219	2.0419	2.1710	1.8530	2.0187	1.7600
$[1/5; 1/5; 3/5; 0; 0]$	0.1500	0.2333	0.9503	1.9628	2.1219	1.7396	1.9348	1.6331
$[1/5; 1/5; 1/5; 2/5; 0]$	0.1833	0.1667	1.3710	2.1819	2.2906	2.0875	2.1703	2.0409
Total	1.0000	1.0000	–	–	–	–	–	–
$\hat{H}_{max}$	2.2906	2.2906	1.5219	2.1819	2.2906	2.0875	2.1703	2.0409
$\hat{H}_{min}$	0.7219	0.7219	0.7219	1.6879	1.9610	1.3153	1.6407	1.1409
$\hat{H}_{max} - \hat{H}_{min}$	1.5687	1.5687	0.8000	0.4940	0.3296	0.7722	0.5296	0.9000
$\frac{\hat{H}_{max} - \hat{H}_{min}}{2}$	1.5063	1.5063	1.1219	1.9349	2.1258	1.7014	1.9055	1.5909

Table 5 allows us to visualize that in general, the maximum estimated value is obtained for the Laplace estimator, $\hat{H}^{Bayes}_{LAP} = 2.2906$, this value being close to the maximum value of the entropy $H_{max} = 2.3219$, for $k = 5$ categories. Also in this table there are values corresponding to the ML estimator that are "close" relatively to the values 1.65 and 1.71 respectively, but these values were calculated for points randomly distributed in [7] and [31] using the estimator ML, $H(P_N) = -\Sigma P_N \ln P_N$.

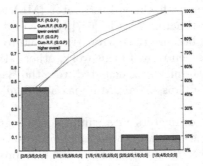

Fig. 4. Pareto diagram of the probability distributions of the number of sides of the Voronoi polygons that appear in the graphical random (DB.2) and clustered (DB.3) passwords.

The probabilities with which these estimators appear only differ significantly in the number of sides with probability $[1/5; 1/5; 3/5; 0; 0]$, since this configuration is more frequent in grouped passwords. Therefore, due to the small sample and because they correspond to approximate probabilities to the entropy estimators, associated with the number of sides of the random graphical passwords and grouped with equal probability, it is not possible to distinguish whether the points are grouped or randomly distributed in said image, as shown in Fig. 4 by the overlap between the probability distributions of the number of sides, which coincides with the result of [6], where they used the maximum plausible estimator to detect symmetry and not it worked. However, in [6] they later used the ML estimator associated with the length of the sides and it was able to distinguish symmetry.

5   Analysis of Results

An important result in this section is that the expected value continues to be approximately 5, regardless of the fact that the points are grouped in a certain region of the study area. Therefore, it is concluded that the characteristic "number of sides of Voronoi polygons" is not able to detect clustering in the graphical passwords of *PassPoint*, on criteria based on expected value and entropy, due to the similarity between the distributions of the number of sides in graphical passwords. Randomized and grouped in *PassPoint*, and due to having a small sample size, since only 5 observations are required (5 polygons in each password).

In our scenario, 300 sets of 5 Voronoi Poisson polygons were simulated in two images of sizes 800×480 and 1366×768 pixels, for an intensity $\lambda = 1.3021 \times 10^{-5}$ and $\lambda = 4.7660 \times 10^{-6}$ respectively. Previous works were generated in a set of the plane 100, 200 and in several iterations of 100,000 to 1,000,000 Voronoi Poisson polygons, with densities $\lambda = 0.16$, unknown and from $\lambda = 178$ until $\lambda = 1,782$ respectively. The known antecedent with the highest number of polygons generated was 208,969,210, but its intensity is unknown. Unlike in previous works, the expected value of the number of sides of the Voronoi polygons in *PassPoint* is 5. In *PassPoint* the number of estimated sides varies in a range from 3 to 7, while its range in previous works is from 3 to 13 by simulation and from 3 to 9 according to the explicit expression of Calka in 2002 [10]. The estimated distribution associated with the number of sides (or vertices) of the Voronoi polygons in previous works was approximated to a generalized three-parameter Gamma distribution, while its distribution in *PassPoint* has not been able to fit any known distribution. The value of the ML estimator associated with the probability distribution of the number of sides of Voronoi Poisson polygons for 200 points in a set of the plane is relatively close to some of the values in *PassPoint*; however, the calculation of the estimators differ on the basis of the logarithms.

6   Conclusions

In this work, the behavior of the number of sides of the Voronoi polygons generated by the graphical passwords of the *PassPoint* graphical authentication system was investigated. Its distribution was estimated, which could not be adjusted to any of the known distributions that the EasyFit program brings by default, including the generalized three-parameter gamma. It was obtained that the expected value of the number of sides of the Voronoi polygons was 5, regardless of the sizes studied. Therefore, the expected value of the number of sides of the Voronoi polygons depends on the number of polygons generated in a study region, and therefore on the intensity, said result differs from that of the antecedents. In the studied scenario, the number of estimated sides varies between 3 and 7, not coinciding with the simulations of the antecedents, in which it varies from 3 to 13. Based on this distribution, a test was proposed, based on the expected value of the number of sides of the polygons, to detect weak graphical passwords formed by grouped points. The effectiveness of the proposed test was evaluated and it was concluded that it is not efficient for the detection of weak graphical passwords of *PassPoint* formed by 5 grouped points. The entropy of the distributions of the number of sides of the Voronoi polygons in random graphical passwords and in weak graphical passwords formed by grouped points was estimated. No significant differences were detected in the value of both entropies. It is concluded that the characteristic number of sides is not effective for the detection of weak graphical passwords of *PassPoint* formed by 5 grouped points. Future work will evaluate the ability of other features of Voronoi polygons, such as the perimeter of a Delaunay triangle and the length of one side of a Voronoi polygon (using the Voronoi entropy associated with this feature) to detect a clustering pattern in *PassPoint*.

References

1. Altay, G., Kurt, Z., Aydinl, N.: Comprehensive review of association estimators for the inference of gene networks. Turkish J. Electr. Eng. Comput. Sci. **24**(3), 695–718 (2016)
2. Aurenhammer, F., Klein, R.: Voronoi diagrams. In: Handbook of Computational Geometry, pp. 201–290. Elsevier Science, Amsterdam (2000)
3. Baddeley, A., Rubak, E., Turner, R.: Spatial Point Patterns: Methodology and Applications with R. CRC Press, Boca Raton (2015). ISBN-13:978-1-4822-2021-7
4. Bhanushali, A., Mangue, B., Vyas, H., Bhanushali , H., Bhogle, P.: Comparison of graphical password authentication techniques. Int. J. Comput. Appl. **116**(1), 0975–8887 (2015)
5. Boots, B.N.: Voronoi (Thiessen) Polygons. Published by Geo Books, ISSN 0306 6142 (1996)
6. Bormashenko, E.: Characterization of Self-Assembled 2D Patterns with Voronoi Entropy (2018). https://doi.org/10.3390/e20120956
7. Bormashenko, E., Legchenkova, I., Frenkel, M.: Symmetry and Shannon Measure of Ordering: Paradoxes of Voronoi Tessellation (2019)
8. Brakke, K.A.: 200,000,000 Random Voronoi Polygons (2015)
9. Brehcist, J.L., Herrera, J.: Mejoras de un sistema de contraseñas gráficas, Universitat Autònoma de Barcelona, Máster interuniversitario de Seguridad de las tecnologías de la información y las comunicaciones (2014)
10. Calka, P.: The explicit expression of the distribution of the number of sides of the typical Poisson Voronoi cell. Preprint of LaPCS, 02 Feb 2002
11. Chiu, S.N.: Spatial point pattern analysis by using Voronoi diagrams and Delaunay tessellations - a comparative study. Biometr. J. **45**(3), 367–376 (2003)
12. Contreras, L., Legón, C.M., Madarro, E., Socorro, R: Estimación de la entropía en sucesiones aleatorias cortas de bytes y bits, Tesis presentada en opción del título de Máster en Ciencias en la Facultad de Matemática y Computación, Instituto de Criptografía, Facultad de Matemática y Computación, Universidad de La Habana (2020)

13. Crain, I.K.: Monte-Carlo simulation of the random Voronoi polygons-preliminary results. Search **3**(5), 220 (1972)
14. Crain, I.K.: The Monte Carlo generation of random polygons. Comput. Geosci. **4**, 131–141 (1978)
15. Dobrin, A.: A review of properties and variations of Voronoi Diagrams. Whitman College (2005). 10.1.1.453.9156
16. Edwards, R., Mardia, K.V., Puri, M.L.: Analysis of central place theory. Bull. Int. Stat. Inst. **47**, 93–110 (1977)
17. Ferraro, M., Zaninetti, L.: On the statistics of area size in two-dimensional thick Voronoi diagrams. Physica A Stat. Mech. Appl. **391**(20), 4575–4582 (2012)
18. Gelfand, A.E., Diggle, P.J., Fuentes, M., Guttorp, P.: Handbook of Spatial Statistics, CRC Press, Boca Raton (2010). ISBN 978-1-4200-7287-7
19. Goodman: Handbook of Discrete and Computational Geometry, 3rd edn. CRC Press (2017). LCCN 2017017843, ISBN 9781498711395
20. Hayen, A., Quine, M.: The proportion of triangles in a Poisson-Voronoi tessellation of the plane. Adv. Appl. Prob. (SGSA) **32**, 67–74 (2002a)
21. Hayen, A., Quine, M.: Calculating the proportion of triangles in a Poisson-Voronoi tessellation of the plane. J. Stat. Comput. Simul. **67**, 351–358 (2002a)
22. Herrera, J.A., Legón, C.M., Piñeiro, L.R., Sosa, G., Rojas, O.: Effectiveness of spatial randomness test in detection of weak graphical passwords in passpoint. In: 4th EAI Internacional conference on Computer Science and Engineering in Health Services (COMPSE 2020) (2020)
23. Hinde, A.L., Miles, R.E.: Monte Carlo estimates of the distributions of the random polygons of the Voronoi tessellation with respect to a Poisson process. J. Stat. Comput. Simul. **10**, 205–223 (1980)
24. Icke, V., Van de Weygaert, R.: Fragmenting the universe. Astron. Astrophys. **184**(1–2) (1987). ISSN 0004–6361
25. Kenkel, N.C., Hoskins, J.A., Hoskins, W.D.: Edge effects in the use of area polygons to study competition. Ecology **70**(1), 272–274 (1989)
26. Kirovski, D., Jodic, N., Roberts, P: Click Passwords, Microsoft Research, One Microsoft Way, Redmond, WA 98052, USA (2020)
27. Komanduri, S., Hutchings, D.R.: Order and entropy in picture passwords. In: Graphics Interface Conference 2008, Windsor, Ontario, Canada (2008)
28. Kumar, S., Kurtz, S.K.: Properties of a two-dimensional Poisson-Voronoi tesselation: a Monte-Carlo study. Mater. Charact. **31**(1), 55–68 (1993)
29. Lashkari A.H., Salleh, R.: A new algorithm for graphical user authentication based on rotation and resizing, A thesis submitted for the master of Computer Science in Data Communication and Computer Networking, Faculty of Computer Science and Information Technology, University Malaya (2010)
30. Lembach, S., Gebert, J.R.: Voronoi and Delaunay diagrams, Technische Universitat Munchen (2010)
31. Limalle, A.V., Narhe, R.D., Dhote, A.M., Ogale, S.B.: Evidence for convective effects in breath figure formation on volatile fluid surfaces. Phys. Rev. Lett. **76**(20), 3762–3765 (1996)
32. Liu, B., Meng, Q., Holstein, H.: Point pattern matching and applications - a review. IEEE Xplore (2003). https://doi.org/10.1109/ICSMC.2003.1243901
33. Miles, R.E.: On the elimination of edge-effects in planar sampling. In: Harding, E.F., Kendall, D.G. (eds.) Stochastic Geometry, pp. 228–247. Wiley, London (1970)
34. Møller, J.: Lectures on Random Voronoi Tessellations. LNS. Springer, New York (1994). https://doi.org/10.1007/978-1-4612-2652-9

35. Muche, L.: Distributional properties of the three-dimensional Poisson Delaunay cell. J. Stat. Phys. **84**, 147–167 (1996)
36. Mumm, M.: Voronoi diagrams. Math. Enthusiast **1**(2) (2004). Article 4
37. Nakoinz, O., Knitter, D.: Modelling Human Behaviour in Landscapes. Springer, Switzerland (2016). https://doi.org/10.1007/978-3-319-29538-1
38. Okabe, A., Boots, B., Sugihara, K., Chiu, S.N.: Spatial tessellations: Concepts and Applications of Voronoi Diagrams (2000). ISBN 0-471-98635-6. British Library Cataloguing in Publication Data
39. Ozcan, M., Yaman, U.: A continuous path planning approach on Voronoi diagrams for robotics and manufacturing applications. In: 29th International Conference on Flexible Automation and Intelligent Manufacturing (FAIM 2019), 24–28 June, Limerick, Ireland (2019)
40. Rittenhouse, R.G., Chaudry, J.A., Lee, M.: Security in graphical authentication. Int. J. Secur. Appl. **7**(3), 347–356 (2013)
41. Rodríguez, O., Legón, C.M., Socorro, R.: Seguridad y usabilidad de los esquemas y técnicas de autenticación gráfica, revista cubana de Ciencias Informáticas, vol. 12, no. Especial UCIENCIA, 13–27 (2018)
42. Schittkowski, K. (2000): EASY-FIT: A Software System for Data Fitting in Dynamical Systems
43. Schittkowski, K.: Data Fitting in Dynamical Systems with EASY-FIT -User's Guide (2002)
44. Schmid, C., Leitner, M.: Monte-Carlo simulation of two-dimensional grain growth (2011)
45. Snibbe, S.S., Tamassia, R.: Introduction to Voronoi diagrams. In: Computational Geometry, C.S. vl. 252 (1993)
46. Tanemura, M.: Statistical distributions of Poisson Voronoi cells in two and three dimensions. FORMA-TOKYO **18**(4), 221–247 (2003)
47. Tico, M., Rusu, C.: Point Pattern Matching using a Genetic Algorithm and Voronoi Tessellation. Tampere University of Technology, Signal Processing Laboratory (1998)
48. Wiedenbeck, S., Waters, J., Birget, J.C., Brodskly, A., Memon, N.: Passpoints: design and longitudinal evaluation of a graphical password system. Int. J. Hum Comput Stud. **63**(1–2), 102–127 (2005)

Modeling Nanocomposites with Ellipsoidal and Conical Inclusions by Optimized Packing

T. Romanova[1,2]([⊠]) [iD], A. Pankratov[1,2] [iD], I. Litvinchev[3] [iD], and E. Strelnikova[4] [iD]

[1] Department of Mathematical Modeling and Optimal Design, Institute for Mechanical Engineering Problems of the National Academy of Sciences of Ukraine, 2/10, Pozharsky Str., Kharkiv 61046, Ukraine
tarom27@yahoo.com
[2] Department of System Engineering, Kharkiv National University of Radioelectronics, 14 Nauky ave., Kharkiv 61166, Ukraine
[3] Graduate Program in Systems Engineering, Nuevo Leon State University (UANL), Monterrey, Av. Universidad s/n, Col. Ciudad Universitaria, 66455 San Nicolas de los Garza, Nuevo Leon, Mexico
[4] Department of Hydroaeromechanics of Power Machines, Institute for Mechanical Engineering Problems of the National Academy of Sciences of Ukraine, 2/10, Pozharsky Str., Kharkiv 61046, Ukraine

Abstract. In this work mathematical models of 3D representative volume elements (RVE) with systems of nanoinclusions are developed. Ellipsoidal and conical nanoinclusions of different sizes are considered in a cuboidal matrix of nanocomposites. Optimized packing is used for computational modeling of filling a given matrix with ellipsoidal and conical nanoinclusions. The proposed approach permits designing different nanoscale structures with desired properties.

Keywords: Ellipsoidal and conical nanoinclusions · Representative volume element · Packing · Phi-function technique

1 Introduction

Solid-type nanocomposites have remarkable mechanical properties and are widely used in practice in many engineering structures and systems. Taking into account diversity of material components and distribution of particles, variety of shapes and arrangements of nanoinclusions, developing new models and methods to study nanocomposites is extremely important.

Computational experiment permits a unified parameterization of elastic properties of nanocomposites in a wide spectrum of their material characteristics, geometric and surface features. Moreover, numerical simulation can replace the expensive field work and essentially reduce the scope, cost and time for experiments.

In contrast to broad experimental studies of nanocomposites and metamaterials [1–3], only a limited number of works on their static and dynamic behavior is known

© ICST Institute for Computer Sciences, Social Informatics and Telecommunications Engineering 2021
Published by Springer Nature Switzerland AG 2021. All Rights Reserved
J. A. Marmolejo-Saucedo et al. (Eds.): COMPSE 2020, LNICST 359, pp. 201–210, 2021.
https://doi.org/10.1007/978-3-030-69839-3_14

[4–7]. The reason is complexity of mathematical models used to describe adequately elastic properties of involved structures. In many cases these models are based on merging basic theoretical principles of continuum mechanics with molecular level descriptions. Computational nanotechnology focuses on numerical simulation in the area [4] and the results are basically related to two-dimensional configurations of the objects [8, 9].

Concerning three-dimensional configurations, they have been analyzed mainly with the assumptions of canonical single spherical particles in the nanocomposite or spherical inclusions in the periodically structured nanomaterial. In this study we consider 3D nanocomposites. Under linear elasticity assumptions, elastic and mechanical properties of composite materials and nanocomposites are considered. The non-classical boundary conditions on the interfaces are addressed to the problems [10–12]. Boundary element methods are applied to numerical solutions of the problems under consideration. The effective algorithm based on Gauss formula is proposed for the singular integrals [13, 14]. A numerical solution of the boundary integral equations is proposed with unknowns distributed on the interface surfaces only. To study size influences at micro-and-nanoscale, the Gurtin-Murdoch theory is applied for the description of nanoscale contacts between the matrix and inclusions. This results in non-classical boundary conditions at the interface surface. This surface is considered as an elastic membrane under a given surface tension and with its own elastic characteristics such as the Lame coefficients [3, 15]. The three-dimensional isotropic elasticity equations are used for Somigliana's identity [1, 16].

In what follows a cube matrix with inhomogeneity inclusions is considered. The inhomogeneities may have the form of an ellipsoid or a (truncated) cone. A representative volume element (RVE) defined by the cube matrix containing non-homogenic elements can be used to study mechanical properties of composites and nano-composites [11, 17].

In [11] expressions for integral operators were obtained, while in [13] and [3] the effective methods were elaborated for numerical integration of corresponding equations. In [3] an effective procedure was presented for estimating the effective modules of nanocomposites. Different types of inclusions were considered resulting in new nanomaterials.

Mathematical and computational models for estimating the effective modulus of nanocomposites using RVE with different mechanical and geometrical characteristics are presented in this paper. To analyze interactions of nanoinclusions in composite materials, 3D optimized packing models are used (see, e.g. [18–27]).

In the current research the phi-function technique (see, e.g. [28–34]) is used to describe placement conditions in mathematical models of filling a given volume with ellipsoidal and conical shaped nanoinclusions.

The structure of the paper is as follows. An optimized packing problem for 3D nanoinclusions and its mathematical model are presented in Sect. 2 together with modeling geometric tools. Solution strategy and computational results are given in Sect. 3, while Sect. 4 presents concluding remarks.

2 Problem Formulation

The following notations are used to formulate the packing problem. Let Ω be a cuboid of having length l, width w and height h, which are considered as variable parameters.

Let a set of nanoinclusions $\{T_i, i \in I_n = \{1, 2, \ldots, n\}\}$ has to be placed completely inside the cuboid Ω without overlaps. Each nanoinclusion T_i can take the shape of an ellipsoid or a truncated cone.

The size of each nanoinclusion T_i is assumed to be fixed. Each nanoinclusion T_i is described in a local coordinate system while a fixed coordinate system is used for the domain Ω.

The arrangement and orientation of T_i are represented by a vector (v_i, θ_i). Here the translation is defined by $v_i = (x_i, y_i, z_i)$ and rotation is represented by the vector θ_i, where $\theta_i = (\theta_i^1, \theta_i^2, \theta_i^3)$, $\theta_i^1, \theta_i^2, \theta_i^3$ are Euler angles. The nanoinclusion T_i, translated by the vector v_i and rotated by θ_i, is stated as

$$T_i(u_i) = \{p \in R^3 : p = v_i + M(\theta_i) \cdot p^0, \forall p^0 \in T_i^0\},$$

where T_i^0 is the nanoinclusion T_i without translation and rotation, $M(\theta_i)$ is a standart rotation matrix.

The problem of filling nanoinclusions into the volume can be stated as the following optimization problem:

Pack all 3D objects $T_i(u_i)$, $i \in I_n$ fully inside the cuboid Ω of minimal volume.

The following constraints have to be met in the problem:

non-overlapping nanoinclusions

$$\text{int } T_i(u_i) \cap \text{int } T_j(u_j) = \varnothing \text{ for } j > i \in I_n, \tag{1}$$

containment of nanoinclusions into the cuboid Ω

$$T_i(u_i) \subset \Omega \Leftrightarrow \text{int } T_i(u_i) \cap \text{int } \Omega^* = \varnothing \text{ for } i \in I_n, \tag{2}$$

where $\Omega^* = R^3 \backslash \text{int}\Omega$.

To describe placement constraints (1)–(2) the phi-functions and quasi-phi-functions are used.

A quasi phi-function for two 3D objects $T_i(u_i)$ and $T_j(u_j)$ is used to present the non-overlapping conditions (1).

Let $P(u_P) = \{(x, y, z): \psi_P = \alpha \cdot x + \beta \cdot y + \gamma \cdot z + \mu_P \leq 0\}$ be a half-space, where $\alpha = \sin\theta_{yP}$, $\beta = -\sin\theta_{xP} \cdot \cos\theta_{yP}$, $\gamma = \cos\theta_{xP} \cdot \cos\theta_{yP}$ and $u_P = (\theta_{xP}, \theta_{yP}, \mu_P)$.

A continuous function defined by

$$\Phi'_{ij}(u_i, u_j, u_P) = \min\{\Phi^{T_iP}(u_i, u_P), \Phi^{T_jP^*}(u_j, u_P)\}, \tag{3}$$

is a quasi-phi-function for $T_i(u_i)$ and $T_j(u_j)$, where

$\Phi^{T_iP}(u_i, u_P)$ is the normalized phi-function for $T_i(u_i)$ and $P(u_P)$ is a half-space, while $\Phi^{T_jP^*}(u_j, u_P)$ is the normalized phi-function for $T_j(u_j)$ and $P^*(u_P) = R^3 \backslash \text{int } P(u_P)$.

As follows from the definition of a quasi-phi-function $\max\limits_{u_P} \Phi'_{ij}(u_i, u_j, u_P)$ is a phi-functions of $T_i(u_i)$ and $T_j(u_j)$ and hence (1) holds if $\max\limits_{u_P} \Phi'_{ij}(u_i, u_j, u_P) \geq 0$.

It follows from the properties of a quasi-phi-function that if $\Phi'_{ij}(u_i, u_j, u_P) \geq 0$ for some u_P, then int $T_i(u_i) \cap$ int $T_j(u_j) = \varnothing$.

To describe containment constraints (2) a phi-function for the objects $T_i(u_i)$ and Ω^* is constructed. This phi-function may be defined in the following form

$$\Phi^{T_i \Omega^*}(l, w, h, u_i) = \min\{\varphi_{ki}(l, w, h, u_i), k = 1, \ldots, 6\}, \tag{4}$$

where $\varphi_{ki}(l, w, h, u_i)$ is a phi-function for $T_i(u_i)$ and a half-space $P_k = \{(x, y, z): \varphi_k \leq 0\}$, while $\varphi_k = 0$ for $k = 1, \ldots, 6$ are equations of sides of the cuboid Ω.

Quasi-phi-Function to Assure Non-overlapping Ellipsoids

Let $T_i(u_i)$ and $T_j(u_j)$ be two ellipsoids defined by corresponding semi-axes $a_i, b_i, c_i = b_i$ and $a_j, b_j, c_j = b_j$.

To describe the non-overlapping condition int $T_i(u_i) \cap$ int $T_j(u_j) = \varnothing$ in (1), a new quasi-phi-function is introduced for ellipsoids $T_i(u_i)$ and $T_j(u_j)$ in the form

$$\Phi'_{ij}(u_i, u_j, u'_{ij}) = n_{ij} \cdot (v_i^T - v_j^T) - \left\| Q^{-1}(\theta_j) \cdot \tau_j \cdot n_{ij}^T \right\| - \left\| Q^{-1}(\theta_i) \cdot \tau_i \cdot n_{ij}^T \right\|,$$

where $\tau_i = \begin{pmatrix} a_i & 0 & 0 \\ 0 & b_i & 0 \\ 0 & 0 & b_i \end{pmatrix}$, $\tau_j = \begin{pmatrix} a_j & 0 & 0 \\ 0 & b_j & 0 \\ 0 & 0 & b_j \end{pmatrix}$,

$v_i = (x_i, y_i, z_i)$, $v_j = (x_j, y_j, z_j)$, $u'_{ij} = (\theta^1_{ij}, \theta^2_{ij})$.

Values n_{ij} and $\theta^1_{ij}, \theta^2_{ij}$ are defined in the following way. A plane $L_{ij} = \{(x, y, z): \alpha_{ij} \cdot x + \beta_{ij} \cdot y + \gamma_{ij} \cdot z + \zeta_{ij} = 0\}$ is constructed for each pair of ellipsoids. The normal vector of the plane L_{ij} is denoted by $n_{ij} = (\alpha_{ij}, \beta_{ij}) = Q(\theta_{ij})(1, 0, 0)^T$, where $Q(\theta_{ij}) = Q_2(\theta^2_{ij}) \cdot Q_1(\theta^1_{ij})$, $\alpha_{ij} = \cos\theta^1_{ij} \cdot \cos\theta^2_{ij}$, $\beta_{ij} = \cos\theta^1_{ij} \cdot \sin\theta^2_{ij}$, $\gamma_{ij} = -\sin\theta^1_{ij}$ and $\theta^1_{ij}, \theta^2_{ij}$ are angles of rotation around the OY and OZ for the plane. Thus, $L_{ij}(\theta^1_{ij}, \theta^2_{ij}, \zeta_{ij}) = \{p = (x, y, z) : n_{ij} \cdot p^T + \zeta_{ij} = 0\}$. Detailed description of the quasi-phi-functions is presented in [30, 33].

Quasi-phi-Function for Non-overlapping Truncated Cones

Each truncated cone is defined by three vectors $p_{i1} = (x_{i1}, y_{i1}, z_{i1})$, $p_{i2} = (x_{i2}, y_{i2}, z_{i2})$ and $\mathbf{n}_i = (n_i^x, n_i^y, n_i^z)$, as well as a pair of parameters r_{i1} and r_{i2}. Here the bottom and top bases of T_i are centred at p_{i1}, p_{i2} and have radii r_{i1}, r_{i2} correspondingly, $\mathbf{n}_i$ denotes the unit vector normal to the bottom (top) base of T_i. For each circular truncated cone $r_{i1} \neq r_{i2}$ and $r_{i1} > 0$, $r_{i2} > 0$. The height of T_i is denoted by h_i.

A quasi phi-function for truncated cones $T_i(u_i)$ and $T_j(u_j)$ is defined in the form

$$\Phi'_{ij}(u_q, u_g, u'_{ij}) = \min\{\Phi_i(u_i, u'_{ij}), \Phi_j^*(u_j, u'_{ij})\},$$

where $\Phi_i(u_i, u'_{ij})$ is a phi-function corresponding to the object $T_i(u_i)$ and the semi-space $\tilde{P}_{ij}$, $\Phi_j^*(u_j, u'_{ij})$ is a phi-function corresponding to the object $T_j(u_i)$ and the semi-space

$\tilde{P}_{ij}^* = R^3 \backslash \text{int } \tilde{P}_{ij}$. Here the vector $u'_{ij} = (\theta^1_{ij}, \theta^2_{ij}, \mu_{ij})$ contains all auxiliary variables of the quasi phi-function Φ^{prime}_{ij} (see [30] for details).

The phi-function corresponding to the object $T_j(u_i)$ and a semi-space $\tilde{P}_{ij}^*$ has the form

$$\Phi_j^*(u_i, u'_{ij}) = \min\{f_1(u_i, u'_{ij}), f_2(u_i, u'_{ij})\},$$

$$f_1(u_i, u'_{ij}) = -\tilde{\mathbf{n}}_{ij} \cdot \tilde{p}_{j1} - \mu_{ij} - r_{j1}\sqrt{1 - (\tilde{\mathbf{n}}_{ij} \cdot \tilde{\mathbf{n}}_i)^2}$$

$$f_2(u_j, u'_{ij}) = -\tilde{\mathbf{n}}_{ij} \cdot \tilde{p}_{j2} - \mu_{ij} - r_{j2}\sqrt{1 - (\tilde{\mathbf{n}}_{ij} \cdot \tilde{\mathbf{n}}_i^q)^2}$$

The non-overlapping condition (1) can be represented by the inequality $\Phi'_{ij}(u_i, u_j, u'_{ij}) \geq 0$.

All variables of the problem can be grouped in the following vector: $u = (l, w, h, u_1, u_2, \dots, u_n, \tau) \in R^\sigma$, where (l, w, h) is the vector of the dimensions of the container Ω; $u_i = (v_i, \theta_i) = (x_i, y_i, z_i, \theta^1_i, \theta^2_i, \theta^3_i)$ represents placement parameters for the object T_i, $i \in I_n$; τ denotes the vector of auxiliary variables u'_{ij} for $j > i \in I_n$.

The optimized packing problem may be formulated in the form

$$\min \kappa(u) \quad \text{s.t. } u \in W, \tag{5}$$

$$W = \{u \in R^\sigma: \Phi'_{ij}(u_i, u_j, u'_{ij}) \geq 0, j > i \in I_n, \Phi_i(l, w, h, u_i) \geq 0, i \in I_n\}, \tag{6}$$

where $\kappa(u) = l \cdot w \cdot h$, $\Phi'_{ij}(u_i, u_j, u'_{ij})$, $\Phi'_{ij}(u_i, u_j, u'_{ij})$ is the quasi phi-function (3) defined for the pair of the 3D objects T_i and T_j (describing the non-intersection constraint (1)), $\Phi_i(l, w, h, u_i)$ is the phi-function (4) for the 3D object $T_i(u_i)$ and the object $\Omega^* = R^3 \backslash \text{int } \Omega$ (enforcing the containment constraint (2)).

Each inequality in (6) contains the phi-function and in fact is a system of inequalities involving differentiable functions. The model (5)–(6) is a continuous nonlinear non-convex programming problem. The formulation (5)–(6) is exact in the sense that it contains all solutions for the original packing problem.

3   Solution Strategy and Computational Results

The solution approach is proposed involving the main stages as follows:

Stage 1. Generating starting points feasible to (5)–(6). The homothetic transformations of objects are used to construct feasible solutions as follows. First, construct a sufficiently large container and circumscribe each nanoinclusion (3D object) by the sphere. Then randomly generate in the large container n centers for the spheres. Scale all the spheres to the full size by solving an auxiliary nonlinear programming subproblem. Form a vector of feasible translation for all nanoinclusions (3D objects). Randomly generate parameters of rotation for all 3D objects. Construct a point feasible to the problem (5)–(6) (see, e.g. [32–34] for details).

Stage 2. Minimize (locally) in the problem (5)–(6) starting from the feasible points generated at Stage 1. Here the optimization procedure described in [35] for large-scale packing problems is used. This algorithm substitutes the original problem (5)–(6) with $O(n2)$ constraints for a sequential solution of nonlinear subproblems with ($O(n)$) nonlinear constraints and variables (see [32, 33] for more details).

Stage 3. The best local minimum obtained at Stage 2 is considered as a solution to the original problem (5)–(6).

Two problem instances below illustrate the work of the proposed multistart approach. The algorithms were implemented and executed on an AMD Athlon 64 X2 5200+ computer. For NLP subproblems the IPOPT solver (https://github.com/coin-or/Ipopt) was used [36]. The sizes of the objects were defined similar to [17].

Example 1. Packing conical nanoinclusions (truncated cones):

a) $n = 35$ including 10 items with $h = 3$ nm, $r_1 = 1.2$ nm, $r_2 = 1$ nm and 25 items with $h = 2$, $r_1 = 0.6$, $r_2 = 0.5$.

The best objective function value obtained for 962.43 s. (10 starting points) is

$$\kappa(u^*) = l^* \cdot w^* \cdot h^* = 8.793475 * 6.162114 * 5.351081 = 289.95579091634.$$

b) $n = 40$ including 10 items with $h = 3$ nm, $r_1 = 1.5$ nm, $r_2 = 1$ nm and 30 items with $h = 2$, $r_1 = 0.8$, $r_2 = 0.5$.

The best objective function value found for 1187.06 s. (10 starting points) is

$$\kappa(u^*) = l^* \cdot w^* \cdot h^* = 7.579022 * 6.926660 * 7.369393 = 386.87329797418.$$

The local optimal solutions corresponding to Example 1 are shown in Fig. 1.

Example 2. Packing $n = 100$ ellipsoidal nanoinclusions (spheroids) with semi axes a = 5 nm, b = 3 nm and c = 3 nm.

The best objective function value found for 35548.86 s. (25 starting points) is

$$\kappa(u^*) = l^* \cdot w^* \cdot h^* = 67.982988 * 71.036815 * 61.835043 = 298619.6603799.$$

The local optimal solution for Example 2 is presented in Fig. 2.

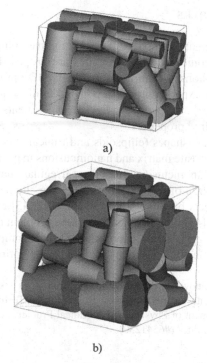

a)

b)

Fig. 1. Local optimal packings for conical nanoinclusions: a) $n = 35$; b) $n = 40$.

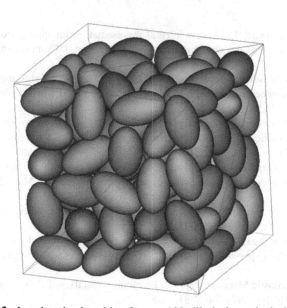

Fig. 2. Local optimal packing for $n = 100$ elliptical nanoinclusions.

4 Concluding Remarks

In this work novel mathematical models of representative volume elements with different mechanical and geometrical characteristics are proposed. To represent mutual interactions of nanoinclusions in composite materials, 3D optimized packing models are developed. Numerical experiment was conducted to illustrate the approach. Using numerical modeling instead of expensive full-scale experiments facilitates synthesis of nanocomposites with desired properties.

Simple convex (regular) shapes (ellipsoids and truncated cones) were used in this work to represent the composite matrix and nanoincusions in packing models. However, in many practical cases nanoinclusions may have irregular shapes [37–41] or can be represented as a composition of regular shapes [37]. An alternative research direction is covering complex objects by more simple shapes [42, 43] or applying other ideas for placement conditions [44]. Large dimension of the problem (5)-(6) may complicate its direct solution. Using aggregation approach [45] or decomposition [46] may help constructing low-dimensional models to get reasonable suboptimal solutions.

Acknowledgment. T. Romanova, A. Pankratov and E. Strelnikova acknowledge partial support by the "Program for the State Priority Scientific Research and Technological (Experimental) Development of the Department of Physical and Technical Problems of Energy of the National Academy of Sciences of Ukraine" (#6541230).

References

1. Barnett, A., Greengard, L.: A new integral representation for quasiperiodic fields and its application to two-dimensional band structure calculations. J. Comput. Phys. **2**, 6898–6914 (2010)
2. Kushch, V., Mogilevskaya, S., Stolarski, H., Crouch, S.: Elastic fields and effective moduli of particulate nanocomposites with the Gurtin-Murdoch model of interfaces. Int. J. Solids Struct. **50**, 1141–1153 (2013)
3. Mykhas'kiv, V., Stasyuk, B.: Effective elastic properties of 3D composites with short curvilinear fibers: numerical simulation and experimental validation. Solid State Phenomena **258**, 452–455 (2017)
4. Mykhas'kiv, V., Zhbadynskyi, I., Zhang, Ch.: Dynamic stresses due to time-harmonic elastic wave incidence on doubly periodic array of penny-shaped cracks. J. Math. Sci. **203**, 114–122 (2014)
5. Miller, R., Shenoy, V.: Size-dependent elastic properties of nanosized structural elements. Nanotechnology **11**, 139–147 (2000)
6. Sigalas, M., Kushwaga, M., Economou, E., Kafesaki, M., Psarobas, I., Steurer, W.: Classical vibrational modes in phononic lattices: theory and experiment. Z. Kristallogr. **220**, 765–809 (2005)
7. Deymier, P.: Acoustic Metamaterials and Phononic Crystals, vol. 7. Springer, Berlin (2013). https://doi.org/10.1007/978-3-642-31232-8
8. Matus, V., Kunets, Y., Mykhas'kiv, V., Boström, A., Zhang, Ch.: Wave propagation in 2D elastic composites with partially debonded fibers by the null field approach. Waves Random Complex Media **19**, 654–669 (2009)

9. Fang, X., Zhang, L., Liu, J.: Dynamic stress concentration around two interacting coated nanowires with surface/interface effect. Meccanica **48**, 287–296 (2013)
10. Gnitko, V., Degtyarev, K., Naumenko, V., Strelnikova, E.: Coupled BEM and FEM analysis of fluid-structure interaction in dual compartment tanks. Int. J. Comput. Methods Exp. Meas. **6**(6), 976–988 (2018)
11. Gnitko, V., Degtyarev, K., Karaiev, A., Strelnikova, E.: Multi-domain boundary element method for axisymmetric problems in potential theory and linear isotropic elasticity. Int. J. Comput. Methods Exp. Meas. WIT Trans. Eng. Sci. **122**, 13–25 (2019)
12. Gnitko, V., Degtyariov, K., Naumenko, V., Strelnikova, E.: BEM and FEM analysis of the fluid-structure interaction in tanks with baffles. Int. J. Comput. Methods Exp. Meas. **5**(3), 317–328 (2017)
13. Gnitko, V., Degtyarev, K., Karaiev, A., Strelnikova, E.: Multi-domain boundary element method for axisymmetric problems in potential theory and linear isotropic elasticity. WIT Trans. Eng. Sci. **122**, 13–25 (2019)
14. Kushch, V., Sevostianov, I.: Effective elastic moduli of a particulate composite in terms of the dipole moments and property contribution tensors. Int. J. Solids Struct. **53**, 1–11 (2015)
15. Kushch, V.: Elastic fields and effective stiffness tensor of spheroidal particle composite with imperfect interface. Mech. Mater. **124**, 45–54 (2018)
16. Dong, C.: Boundary element analysis of nanoinhomogeneities of arbitrary shapes with surface and interface effects. Eng. Anal. Boundary Elem. **35**, 996–1002 (2011)
17. Mirkhalaf, S., Andrade Pires, F., Simoes, R.: Determination of the size of the Representative Volume Element (RVE) for the simulation of heterogeneous polymers at finite strains. Finite Elem. Anal. Des. **119**, 30–44 (2016)
18. Strelnikova, E., et al.: Optimized packings in analysis of 3D nanocomposites with inclusion systems. In: 2020 IEEE KhPI Week on Advanced Technology (KhPIWeek), Kharkiv, Ukraine, pp. 377–381 (2020). https://doi.org/10.1109/KhPIWeek51551.2020.9250142
19. Burtseva, L., Valdez Salas, B., Romero, R., Werner, F.: Recent advances on modelling of structures of multi-component mixtures using a sphere packing approach. Int. J. Nanotechnol. **13**, 44–59 (2016)
20. Liu, X., Liu, J., Cao, A., Yao, Z.: HAPE3D – a new constructive algorithm for the 3D irregular packing problem. Front. Inf. Technol. Electron. Eng. **16**(5), 380–390 (2015)
21. Duriagina, Z., Lemishka, I., Litvinchev, I., et al.: Optimized filling of a given cuboid with spherical powders for additive manufacturing. J. Oper. Res. Soc. China (2020). https://doi.org/10.1007/s40305-020-00314-9
22. Pintér, J., Kampas, F., Castillo, I.: Globally optimized packings of non-uniform size spheres in R^d: a computational study. Optim. Lett. **12**(3), 585–613 (2018)
23. Gately, R., in het Panhuis, M.: Filling of carbon nanotubes and nanofibres. Beilstein J. Nanotechnol. **6**(1), 508–516 (2015)
24. Mollon, G., Zhao, J.: 3D generation of realistic granular samples based on random fields theory and Fourier shape descriptors. Comput. Methods Appl. Mech. Eng. **279**, 46–65 (2014)
25. Ustach, V., Faller, R.: The raspberry model for protein-like particles: ellipsoids and confinement in cylindrical pores. Eur. Phys. J. Spec. Top. **225**(8–9), 1643–1662 (2016)
26. Wang, X., Zhao, L., Fuh, J.Y.H., Lee, H.P.: Effect of porosity on mechanical properties of 3D printed polymers: experiments and micromechanical modeling based on X-ray computed tomography analysis. Polymers **11**(7), 1154 (2019)
27. Zhao, C., Jiang, L., Teo, K.L.: A hybrid chaos firefly algorithm for three-dimensional irregular packing problem. J. Ind. Manag. Optim. **16**(1), 409–429 (2020)
28. Stoyan, Y., Romanova, T., Pankratov, A., Kovalenko, A., Stetsyuk, P.: Balance layout problems: mathematical modeling and nonlinear optimization. In: Fasano, G., Pintér, J.D. (eds.) Space Engineering. SOIA, vol. 114, pp. 369–400. Springer, Cham (2016). https://doi.org/10.1007/978-3-319-41508-6_14

29. Grebennik, I.V., Kovalenko, A.A., Romanova, T.E., Urniaieva, I.A., Shekhovtsov, S.B.: Combinatorial configurations in balance layout optimization problems. Cybern. Syst. Anal. **54**(2), 221–231 (2018). https://doi.org/10.1007/s10559-018-0023-2

30. Pankratov, A., Romanova, T., Litvinchev, I.: Packing oblique 3D objects. Mathematics **8**(7), 1130 (2020)

31. Stoyan, Y., et al.: Optimized packings in space engineering applications: Part I. In: Fasano, G, Pintér, J.D. (eds.) Modeling and Optimization in Space Engineering. SOIA, vol. 144, pp. 395–437. Springer, Cham (2019). https://doi.org/10.1007/978-3-030-10501-3_15

32. Romanova, T., Bennell, J., Stoyan, Y., Pankratov, A.: Packing of concave polyhedra with continuous rotations using nonlinear optimization. Eur. J. Oper. Res. **268**(1), 37–53 (2018)

33. Romanova, T., Litvinchev, I., Pankratov, A.: Packing ellipsoids in an optimized cylinder. Eur. J. Oper. Res. **285**(2), 429–443 (2020)

34. Romanova, T., et al.: Sparsest balanced packing of irregular 3D objects in a cylindrical container Eur. J. Oper. Res. (2020) https://doi.org/10.1016/j.ejor.2020.09.021

35. Romanova, T., Stoyan, Y., Pankratov, A., Litvinchev, I., Marmolejo, J.A.: Decomposition algorithm for irregular placement problems. In: Vasant, P, Zelinka, I., Weber, G.-W. (eds.) ICO 2019. AISC, vol. 1072, pp. 214–221. Springer, Cham (2020). https://doi.org/10.1007/978-3-030-33585-4_21

36. Wächter, A., Biegler, L.T.: On the implementation of an interior-point filter line-search algorithm for large-scale nonlinear programming. Math. Program. **106**(1), 25–57 (2006)

37. Leao, A.A., Toledo, F.M., Oliveira, J.F., Carravilla, M.A., Alvarez-Valdés, R.: Irregular packing problems: a review of mathematical models. Eur. J. Oper. Res. **282**, 803–822 (2020)

38. Araújo, L.J., Özcan, E., Atkin, J., Baumers, M.: Analysis of irregular three-dimensional packing problems in additive manufacturing: a new taxonomy and dataset. Int. J. Prod. Res. **57**, 5920–5934 (2018)

39. Wang, S., Marmysh, D., Ji, S.: Construction of irregular particles with superquadric equation in DEM. Theor. Appl. Mech. Lett. **10**, 68–73 (2020)

40. Liu, X., Liu, J.-M., Cao, A.-X., Yao, Z.-L.: HAPE3D—a new constructive algorithm for the 3D irregular packing problem. Front. Inf. Technol. Electron. Eng. **16**, 380–390 (2015)

41. Garboczi, E., Bullard, J.: 3D analytical mathematical models of random star-shape particles via a combination of X-ray computed microtomography and spherical harmonic analysis. Adv. Powder Technol. **28**, 325–339 (2017)

42. Pankratov, A., Romanova, T., Litvinchev, I., Marmolejo-Saucedo, J.A.: An optimized covering spheroids by spheres. Appl. Sci. **10**(5), 1846 (2020)

43. Stoyan, Y., Romanova, T., Scheithauer, G., Krivulya, A.: Covering a polygonal region by rectangles. Comput. Optim. Appl. **48**(3), 675–695 (2011)

44. Litvinchev, I., Romanova, T., Corrales-Diaz, R., Esquerra-Arguelles, A., Martinez-Noa, A.: Lagrangian approach to modeling placement conditions in optimized packing problems. Mobile Netw. Appl. (2020). https://doi.org/10.1007/s11036-020-01556-w

45. Litvinchev, I., Rangel, S.: Localization of the optimal solution and a posteriori bounds for aggregation. Comput. Oper. Res. **26**(10–11), 967–988 (1999)

46. Litvinchev, I., Mata, M., Rangel, S., Saucedo, J.: Lagrangian heuristic for a class of the generalized assignment problems. Comput. Math Appl. **60**(4), 1115–1123 (2010)

Applications in the Education Sector

Design Strategies for University Educational Supply Chain

María del Carmen Toledo Muñoz[1]([✉]) [iD], Rosario Lucero Cavazos Salazar[2] [iD],
and José Mario Valadez Cedillo[1,2] [iD]

[1] Universidad Autónoma de Nuevo León,
San Nicolás de los Garza, Nuevo León, Mexico
mariadelctoledo92@gmail.com, lucero.cavazos@uanl.mx,
mario.valadez@gmail.com
[2] ABC Institute, Rupert-Karls-University Heidelberg, Heidelberg, Germany

Abstract. The University Educational Institutions are currently perceiving an increase in the demand for their services, which forces them to seek strategies that allow them to have well identified the activities to be carried out at each stage of their processes. This study seeks to identify the strategies, methods, and tools that allow the design of the University Educational Supply Chain, based on a systemic review of the literature. Following as a working method the classification of documents by topic of interest, then the characteristics of the university educational supply chain are analyzed, supply chain design tools applied in different environments are analyzed and the most suitable methods are selected based on established criteria. Feasible to apply in the university educational environment. It is obtained as a result of this work that the Supply Chain Operations Reference Model, the Value Stream Mapping, and Simulation, are supply chain design strategies that are adjusted to the university educational environment and that serve as, help to redesign processes, measure the performance and effectiveness of the services and products offered to students, the labor market and society in general

Keywords: University Educational Institutions · Supply chain · University educational supply chain · Supply chain design

1 Introduction

The study of the supply chain currently represents of interest to managers, leaders, and stakeholders of University Educational Institutions [1, 2] who seek to meet the expectations of the labor market and students entering these institutions.

Universities represent the basis for the development of society [3], but they are currently facing phenomena such as the massive increase in the demand for their services, lack of communication between the university education sector and the labor market [4, 5] and the scarce funding available to universities to develop their curricula [5, 6].

J. A. Marmolejo-Saucedo et al. (Eds.): COMPSE 2020, LNICST 359, pp. 213–230, 2021.
https://doi.org/10.1007/978-3-030-69839-3_15

This situation demands an improvement in the administrative processes and operations of the university education sector [5,7], which leads these institutions to incorporate supply chain approaches in their work strategies [8,9].

This work aims to analyze supply chain strategies, methods, and tools that can be integrated to the university education sector and that contribute to meet the increase in demand for university services, strengthen the communication flow between the labor market and university education institutions and serve as sustainability alternatives for the University Education Supply Chain. The structure of this document is as follows: first, a summary of the articles and journals analyzed is made, according to keywords used in the search system, then the supply chain for university educational institutions is defined, the existing strategies and methodologies for the design of the supply chain are analyzed and finally, the best methods are selected to increase the efficiency and effectiveness in the university educational processes.

2   Literature Review

Understanding the background of studies related to the Supply Chain is an important step that allows you to have a vision of the evolution of these concepts over time. Researchers such as [8] show a timeline, which allows us to visualize how supply chain management has transcended and how its applicability has been both in the manufacturing, service, and education areas. The evolution of the concepts can be seen in Fig. 1.

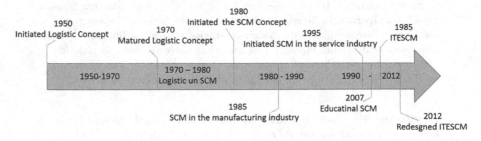

Fig. 1. Evolutionary line of supply chain management. Source: own elaboration with information from [8].

During the 1940s and 1950s, logistics was related to the need of the military to acquire, maintain, and transport all its materials and personnel from one facility to another [8]. Then, in the 1960s and 1970s, studies related to physical distribution and logistics began, incorporating in the 1980s the concept of Supply Chain Management due to the need that manufacturing companies saw to incorporate new organizational functions [10,11]. [8] emphasize that the supply chain is characterized by being seen as a unique entity, where strategic decision making at the top level is necessary to manage the chain in its original formulation.

One of the first authors that proposes to apply supply chain tools in University Educational Institutions is [12], who seeks to join theory with practice and proposes a contingency model, which is achieved by applying a questionnaire to employers and students and which allows establishing improvement strategies for the integration between companies, suppliers and clients of University Educational Institutions.

On the other hand, [13] create a model of supply chain management based on strategies that are implemented in the service and manufacturing industry where the structure of the university educational supply chain is defined.

[11] proposes the first largescale empirical study where he defines that the educational supply chain, the research supply chain and educational management are the necessary elements to apply an Integrated University Educational Supply Chain Management Model.

3   Methodology

The methodology proposed in this study consists of a systemic review of the literature that allows to establish criteria for the selection of one or more supply chain design tools that can be adapted to the characteristics of the university educational supply chain and that also allow establish the configuration of the supply chain processes, determine the level of integration between the processes and that contributes to establishing continuous improvement strategies that allow them to be efficient and able to compete in the increasingly global market.

The methodology for selecting the tools consists of three stages which are shown in Fig. 2 and explained below.

Stage I: This stage begins with a planned review of the documents required for the development of this study, which allows for the selection of studies related to the university educational supply chain and supply chain design strategies.

Stage II: Once the different supply chain design strategies have been identified and the peculiarities of the university educational supply chain have been analyzed, selection criteria are established to identify which of the strategies is best adapted to the type of chain to be designed. At this stage, the different scenarios in which the selected design strategies were implemented, the peculiarity of each supply chain studied, as well as the objectives pursued in each study are considered in order to identify those factors that were most repeated and thus determine a common criterion that allows the selection of one or more tools that best fit the case study.

Stage III: In this stage, an analysis of the results obtained from the previous stage is made, where the selected tool is described, based on the coincidence that exists between the criteria selected in the previous stage, thus establishing a frame of reference from the analysis of case studies that allows the understanding of the applicability of the selected tool in the studied environment.

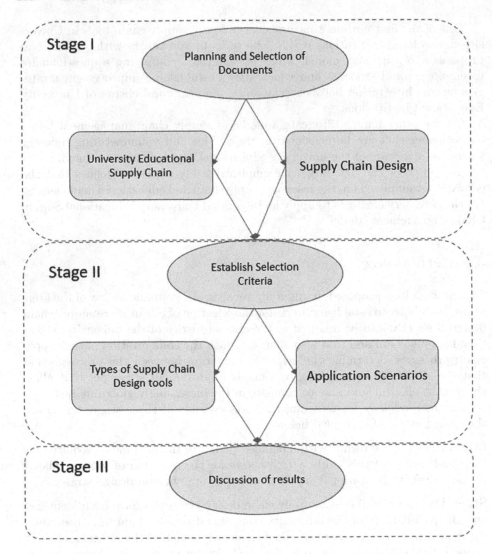

Fig. 2. Methodology for the selection of supply chain design tool criteria. Source: own elaboration.

3.1   Stage I: Planning and Document Review

For the selection of the documents, the following databases were used: Scopus, EBSCO, Web of Science, Elseiver, MIAR, Research Gate, Scielo and Google Scholar. The categories for the search and selection of the documents established were: University Educational Institutions, Supply Chain, Supply Chain in University Educational Institutions, Supply Chain Design and Supply Chain Design Methods and Tools.

A total of 132 articles were selected of which 59 were related to University Educational Institutions, 26 analyzed the general supply chain, 132 analyzed the University Educational Supply Chain, 14 were oriented to the design of the supply chain and 20 of them provided the tools that help in the design of the supply chain. The publication date of these studies is between 2010 and 2018.

The main magazines consulted were Industrial Management and Data Systems; Iberoamerican Business Journal; European Journal of Business and Management; Computers and Industrial Engineering; Competitiveness Review. An International Business Journal; Science, Academic Research and Development; Advances in Decision Sciences; International Journal of Production Research; Industrial Engineering; Management, Technology and Social; Revista Iberoamericana para la Educación; Journal Manufacturing Technology Management; Journal Of Computational Science; International Conference on Industrial Engineering and Operations Management Dhaka; International Journal of Supply Chain Management; Supply Chain Management: An International Journal; Engineering and Development; International Conference on Smart Technologies for Mechanical Engineering; Engineering and Technology; International Journal of Manufacturing Engineering.

From this analysis, it stands out that most of the studies are directed to the analysis of the management and design of the manufacturing supply chain [9,11], only a few analyze this problem in the service industry, where the work of [2,5,8,14] related to the design and management of the supply chain in University Educational Institutions.

Supply Chain in University Educational Institutions. Ensuring development in an increasingly competitive national and international environment implies, for the UIS, considering quality in the teaching and learning processes [3]. For this purpose, the UIS need to adopt supply chain concepts in their own institutions, which contribute to the improvement of productive and service processes, satisfying with quality the expectations of the demanders [2].

The concept of the educational supply chain is a topic that is of interest to many authors [15], since like other supply chains they require the coordination of all their nodes to achieve an aligned flow of information, production and distribution [2].

The University Education Supply Chain is the integrated set of the education supply chain and the research supply chain [8], as shown in Fig. 3. This holistic view of the University Education Supply Chain concept given by [8], shows in a simplified way the twoway sense in which information and service flows, at a single level of supply chain management for universities.

[2], consider that the Educational Supply Chain is characterized by two types of services, one dedicated to teaching, which establishes the direct and indirect services to process inputs; and secondly we have the research services or research projects, considered more expensive and prolonged, requiring a personalized, proactive and reactive supply chain to satisfy the demanders.

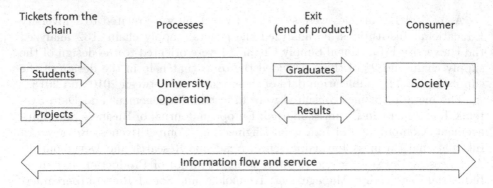

Fig. 3. Holistic view of a University Education Supply Chain. Source: Own elaboration with information of [8].

[16], highlights that the University Education Supply Chain involves schools, colleges of higher education, current students, university staff and employers, who in collaboration with the University Institutions, multilevel and service providers who allow the development of curricula that satisfy the final consumer. Figure 4 shows the twoway flow of the University Education Supply Chain that is achieved through integration between providers, University Institutions and customers.

[2,15] classify the suppliers of the supply chain, according to their entries, considering among them suppliers of teaching services, who become colleges or high schools, universities, faculties within the same university educational institutions, students, family members, organizations that provide scholarships and financial support, suppliers of assets, equipment, and of educational materials such as stationery, technologies, among others [2,15].

[1,11], also establish that project and research providers within the supply chain are selffinanced by the university's own educational institutions and external project providers who provide financial support to universities and research centers.

[9] point out that one of the main objectives of an educational supply chain is to improve the welfare of the final customer, who according to [11] become the students themselves who provide their bodies, minds, belongings, as raw materials needed to obtain graduates and quality research results [11]. On the other hand, [16] considers the labor market, as a client of the University Education Supply Chain, who expect as a result graduates to have the knowledge and skills necessary to perform the work for which they were employed.

To be able to meet market needs and meet customer expectations, University Educational Institutions must have a certain degree of knowledge about the parameters in their supply chains, including suppliers, customers and consumers [9].

The University Educational Institutions must seek the improvement and integration of their processes and services that meet the quality requirements and satisfy the expectations of the demanders, implementing design strategies that

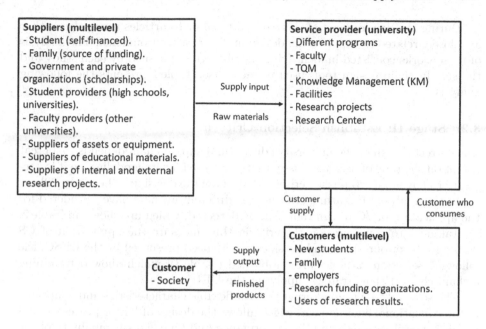

Fig. 4. Integration of information and service flows at each level of the University Education Supply Chain. Source: Own elaboration with information of [16].

allow the university educational institutions to have a much more dynamic and competitive supply chain [2,17].

Through an empirical study conducted at 10 universities in Malaysia, [18] found that CS practices have a high impact on university performance, especially information sharing practices.

Supply Chain Design. Supply chain design is defined as the process of developing, implementing and managing resources, processes and information, which seeks to make the strategic objectives of any institution, company or enterprise achievable over time .

The supply chain design process has been oriented to solve problems related to the location of the facilities, the installed capacity, the current market situation, and the selection of suppliers, among others [20].

The complexity that is perceived in the process of supply chain design is given by the hesitation in selecting the best improvement strategies, the attention of management and the accuracy of cost estimation [20].

[19] suggest that design strategies employed in one supply chain do not generate the same result when applied in another in a different environment. Thus, in the face of the diversity of environments, multiple responses have occurred that contribute to supply chain design techniques and tools [21].

During the development of this work, a total of 14 articles are analyzed that are closely related to supply chain design in different environments. The analysis of these works consisted in identifying the objectives pursued by each study and the supply chain design tools used in each case. Table 1 presents the following analysis.

3.2   Stage II: Establish Selection Criteria

The correct design of the university educational supply chain depends to a great extent on the type of design strategy that is selected for its modeling, so it is necessary to have well established criteria that allow the decision to be made [22].

In the analyzed literature, criteria that different authors have considered for the application of SC design tools can be detected, which are shown in Table 2.

Taking into consideration the criteria that measure the application of CS design tools set out above and considering the need presented by the UESC, the following selection variables are established (Table 3), which allow determining a chain chain design strategy supply for the UEI.

The selected tool is an alternative with flexible characteristics and adaptable to the educational environment, which allows the design of UESC processes, and makes it possible to measure the performance and financial sustainability of the chain, as well as to establish continuous improvement strategies in the whole chain.

3.3   Stage III: Discussion of Results

During the development of this research, CS design methods and tools are identified that can be applied in the EUI due to their flexibility and applicability in different sectors, and that help to redesign the processes in the chain to meet the growing demand for services educational institutions, as well as establishing indicators to measure the performance and quality of the services offered to students, the labor market and society in general.

Among the supply chain design methods that best fit the evaluation criteria established above are the SCOR model, the Value Chain Mapping, and the use of integrated simulation of these two models. Each of these supply chain design tools is described below.

SCOR Model. The Supply Chain Operations Reference Model, or SCOR model, was developed in 1996 by the Supply Chain Council (SCC) to create a standard that enables companies to improve their supply chain operations [23,24].

SCOR can be used to describe anything from simple to complex supply chains, using a common language to describe processes, process performance indicators, improvement practices and technologies [21,25] (Wang, Chan, and Pauleen, 2010; Rashid, and Weston, 2012). Good supply chain management executed under SCOR enables the parties involved to manage, improve their methods and communicate more efficiently and effectively, achieving excellence in the

Table 1. Summary of Supply Chain Design studies and methods. Source: Own Elaboration

Authors	Research objective	Instrument
Rashid Weston (2012)	Create and implement an integrated methodology for the design of complex supply chains	Business model Causal Loop Diagram Simulation
Carvalho et al. (2012)	Improve the resilience of interrupted supply chains by studying alternative scenarios	Simulation
Pardillo-Baez & Gómez-Acosta (2013)	Provide a node design model that contributes to integrated management among the chain's node actors, guaranteeing the required levels of efficiency and effectiveness	Simulation VSM SCOR Model
Prasad, Subbaiah, Rao (2014)	Achieve an integration between competitive and supply chain strategies, based on a supply chain design methodology	Quality function deployment (QFD)
López Manzano et al. (2014)	Improve communication processes and channels in a telecommunications company, based on a redesign of its internal supply chain	Ciclo Deming Modelo DAFO SCOR
Orjuela Castro (2018)	Assess the impact of the type of design of the perishable food supply chain on the balance of logistics flows	Optimization Simulation
Fajardo (2018)	Reduce the delivery time of a company dedicated to the transformation of coated steel sheets in order to meet the delivery deadlines agreed with the client	DMAIC methodology
Carvalho et al. (2010)	Meet the requirements established between the auto parts industry and the automaker, based on a supply chain redesign case study	Data collection and analysis
Hilletofth (2012)	Develop a framework for supply chain design to demonstrate the key benefits and requirements of a differentiated supply chain	Market information gathering
Melnyk et al. (2014)	Understand the three key levels to consider in supply chain design	Case study analysis
Authors	Objectives of the study	Instruments
Masoumik et al. (2014)	Develop a conceptual framework that can shape the components of a sustainable supply chain	Data review and analysis
Pashaei 6 Olhager (2015)	Identify gaps and opportunities for improvement, based on a review of the literature, on the relationship between product architecture and supply chain design	Bibliographic review and analysis
Ivanov et al. (2015)	Analyze recent research on supply chain design with disruption considerations in terms of domino effects	Analyze the literature
Asmussen et al. (2018)	Determine the factors that affect the supply chain design decision making process	Case study analysis

Table 2. Selection criteria of supply chain design instruments. Source: Own Elaboration

Instruments	Selection criteria	Authors
Business model	–It is mainly applicable to complex supply chains –Allows the modeling of the supply chain structure	Rashid, Weston (2012)
Causal loop diagram	–It allows visualizing the behavior of the indicators in the supply chain	Rashid Weston (2012)
Simulation	–Allows you to visualize the behavior of different scenarios in the supply chain –Allows the design of the supply chain network –Contributes to decision-making on improvement strategies –It is flexible and can be applied to all kinds of supply chains	Rashid Weston (2012) Carvalho et al. (2012) Pardillo-Baez & Gómez-Acosta (2013) Orjuela Castro (2018)
Value stream mapping	–Allows the redesign of processes in the supply chain –Allows determining limiting operations –Allows establishing improvement strategies –Flexible and adaptable to any type of supply chain	Pardillo-Baez & Gómez-Acosta (2013)
SCOR model	–Process reengineering –Benchmarking –Measurement of processes –Adaptable to any type of supply chain	Pardillo-Baez & Gómez-Acosta (2013) López Manzano et al. (2014)
Quality function deployment (QFD)	–Allows determining competitive strategies in the supply chain –Allows you to define performance within the supply chain	Prasad Subbaiah, Rao (2014)
Deming cycle	–Allows the establishment of continuous improvement strategies based on the analysis of indicators in the supply chain	López Manzano et al. (2014)
Deming cycle	–Allows the establishment of continuous improvement strategies based on the analysis of indicators in the supply chain	López Manzano et al. (2014)
DAFO analysis	–Analyzes the internal and external environment of the supply chain –Allows the establishment improvement strategies in the supply chain –It is flexible and can be applied to all types supply chains	López Manzano et al. (2014)
Optimization	–Optimizes the development and selection of product, process, services in the supply chain –Allows the alignment of strategy within the supply chain It is flexible and can be applied to all types of supply chains	Orjuela Castro (2018)
DMAIC methodology	–Allows the definition of indicators in the processes of the supply chain –Analyzes and establishes improvement strategy	Fajardo (2018)

Table 3. Selection criteria of supply chain design Instruments. Source: Own elaboration.

	Evaluation criteria				
Instruments	Flexible	Process design	Measurable	Improvement strategy	Number of criteria met
Business model		X			1
Causal loop diagram		X			1
Simulation	X	X		X	3
Value stream mapping	X	X	X	X	4
SCOR model	X	X	X		3
Quality Function Deployment (QFD)			X	X	2
Deming Cycle				X	1
DAFO	X			X	2
Optimization	X	X			2
DMAIC methodology		X		X	2

organizational structure of the value chain and achieving customer satisfaction [24, 26, 27]. SCOR has several valuable contributions, including its contribution of standardized metrics for measuring supply chain performance [28].

The five main management processes (Fig. 5), by which the SCOR model is governed, are Planning (Plan), Procurement (Source), Manufacturing (Make), Distribution (Deliver) and Return [24].

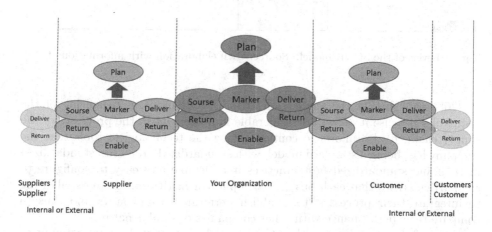

Fig. 5. Structure of the SCOR model. Source: Own elaboration with information of [24].

SCOR includes three levels of detail (Fig. 6), where a) Higher Level. Process Types b) Configuration Level. Categories of Processes and c) Level of Process Elements. Decomposition of the Processes, to these three levels is added a level of implementation which is out of the scope of the scheme, but what is necessary to implement since it allows to define the practices to reach the competitive advantages and thus to adapt to the business conditions [26]. At each of these levels, the supply chain performance indicators are determined, which are divided into five performance attributes: Reliability, Flexibility, Responsiveness, Cost and Assets.

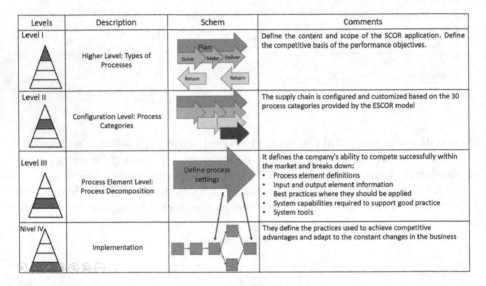

Levels	Description	Schem	Comments
Level I	Higher Level: Types of Processes	Plan, Surce, Make, Deliver, Return, Return	Define the content and scope of the SCOR application. Define the competitive basis of the performance objectives.
Level II	Configuration Level: Process Categories		The supply chain is configured and customized based on the 30 process categories provided by the ESCOR model
Level III	Process Element Level: Process Decomposition	Define process settings	It defines the company's ability to compete successfully within the market and breaks down: • Process element definitions • Input and output element information • Best practices where they should be applied • System capabilities required to support good practice • System tools
Nivel IV	Implementation		They define the practices used to achieve competitive advantages and adapt to the constant changes in the business

Fig. 6. Levels of the SCOR model. Source: Own elaboration with information of [26].

[26] establish that the application of the SCOR model is beneficial for the companies because it allows a considerable improvement in the processes of the supply chain, it also allows to continue using the technological tools that the company has, being a standard model, with standardized processes, standardized metrics and standardized best practices it is flexible and easy to configure to the particularities that each business, company or institution presents, allowing to integrate their processes, to establish performance indicators and thus to compare their performance with other companies of similar nature.

Some of the limitations of the SCOR model are that it does not attempt to describe each Business Process or Activity, and the model does not contemplate what is related to demand generation processes, product development or research and development. And as for the activities of Human Resources, Training, Systems, Administration and Quality Assurance, SCOR does not contemplate them anymore if they should be considered when applying this model [25].

Value Stream Mapping. Value Stream Mapping (VSM) is a Lean Manufacturing management tool, which allows the visualization of all the processes carried out within an organization, showing the current state of the company, identifying its points of improvement and serving as a contribution for comparison during the implementation of any of the lean manufacturing tools [5]. It supports the redesign of processes, seeking to develop efficient and flexible competitive supply chains [29].

This type of method considers three fundamental pillars: continuous improvement (Kaizen), total quality control and just in time (Just in time), with the objective of making the company, institution or enterprise profitable, competitive and efficient [30].

The VSM model works in manufacturing companies, service companies [31] and even in University Educational Institutions [5], allowing to visualize multiple processes, including the flow of material and information within the institution, as well as the level of integration that exists in them, identifying the source of waste that limits the institutions.

[32] points out that the use of VSM could help improve visibility and develop a risk management system.

[5] proposes to apply this model in university educational institutions, based on the 4 stages of the VSM and a series of steps established in each of them, which are shown in Fig. 7.

The application of this method allows for a visual representation that determines where the limiting operations are located, using symbols, metrics and arrows, which make it possible to show and improve the flow of inventory and information required to produce a product or service that is delivered to a consumer.

On the other hand, [5], highlights that some advantages of applying VSM are

- They help to visualize the global process allowing an integral vision that things really work allowing to see events from the client's point of view,
- They allow to see the losses of a process,
- They allow to link the connections between the material and the information flow and,
- They help the alignment of the organization; that is, giving a starting point for the implementation of an improvement while involving people.
- Manifests a link between the flow of information and material.
- Facilitates a common language for the interpretation of manufacturing processes.

On the other hand, [5] highlights some challenges that institutions present when implementing VSM, among them

- Problems when monitoring processes.
- Ignorance of the model by the staff within the institution.
- Little integration between the processes of the entire supply chain.

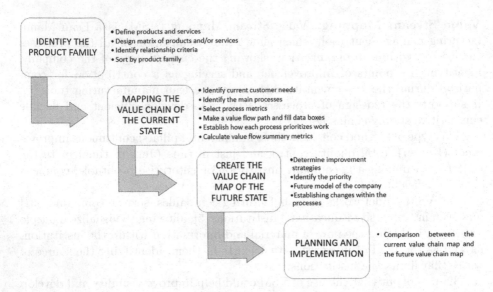

Fig. 7. Value stream mapping model. Source: Own elaboration with information from [5].

- The large number of products and processes that are not yet defined within the institution.
- Wide range of products and production flows that are not yet clearly defined by the institutions.
- Lack of support from top management.

Simulation. Simulation modeling has been widely implemented in many disciplines to replicate and predict behaviors [21], allowing the identification of gaps between actual performance and the current state of the supply chain [33].

Simulation models are often complex in certain cases, since they require coding static and dynamic properties of the systems [21], so it is necessary to have well established the situation being addressed.

According to [34] Simulation is a tool that allows to predict a certain situation in a short period of time, from the consideration of variables that intervene in the modeled scenario, if seeing of support for the election of improvement strategies and for the design of processes in the organizations. In this way, simulation allows to anticipate risks in the supply chains [35].

One of the benefits of simulation is that it is a tool that allows the evaluation of theories and also serves to analyze the organizational situation [36]. [34] considers simulation as a strategy for companies that allows them to reduce the risks that can occur when making a decision in a certain situation in the organization, allowing the reduction of time, costs and helping to visualize the future effects of the implementation of a project [37].

The literature review has shown how the Simulation has been combined with other supply chain design strategies to obtain better results in implementing change and improvement strategies in the organization [21, 27, 33, 37].

Simulation, together with the VSM model, allows us to see in a clearer, faster and more feasible way the limiting operations that affect the current and future state of the value map in the supply chain [37].

On the other hand, it was found in the literature that most of the studies that use simulation in conjunction with the SCOR model focus on solving problems, and apply it fundamentally to the improvement plan process at level 4 of the model, serving as a validation tool for decision making [27].

The truth is that simulation not only makes testing ideas easier, cheaper and faster, but also provides an immediate evaluation of proposed changes in the system [38].

Using simulation models requires appropriate tools such as: SIMUL8 (https://www.simul8.com/), Arena and iThink, among others [21], which provide behavioral analysis capabilities that can predict system results with reference to selected system performance measures

Despite the fact that the application of Simulation allows for a reduction in costs, a decrease in decisionmaking time, and provides greater reliability when selecting improvement strategies, it presents some restrictions such as: the lack of systematization of information, the need to study in detail the relationships between system elements, and the difficulty of integrating and making explicit large models, it facilitates the study of systems, mainly those of smaller sizes and specific phenomena.

4 Conclusions

Although the study of the supply chain is a very frequent topic in industrial and commercial sectors, since it allows to improve the performance of the chain, its application in the educational sector is limited. Several researchers found that there are important opportunities in education systems, such as weak communication between the labor market and universities, lack of funding, and overcrowding. This establishes an interesting avenue of research to analyze educational processes in detail and develop initiatives to redesign their supply chain.

Weak communication between the labor market, students, and the university education supply chain results in a curriculum that is not aligned with the needs of employers, students, and society. Educational institutions require strategies to meet the expectations of their stakeholders.

The literature review also reveals supply chain design strategies that can be applied to University Educational Institutions, among which are considered the Supply Chain Operations Reference Model (SCOR model), the Value Chain Mapping (VSM) and the Simulation.

The implementation of these supply chain design strategies in educational institutions contributes to increase the efficiency and effectiveness of their services and products offered by the different educational institutions.

This study contributes to the knowledge about the use of methods and strategies of university educational supply chain design, a topic that has been little addressed in the literature. Future work could expand to look more deeply at the impact of some of these design models on university educational institutions. This would help to demonstrate that supply chain design strategies contribute to an improvement in their entire supply chain, enabling them to meet the needs of today's market.

References

1. Basu, G., Jeyasingam, J., Habib, M.M.: Education supply chain management model to achieve sustainability in private Universities in Malaysia: a review. Int. J. Supply Chain Manag. **5**(4), 24–37 (2016)
2. Ortega Jiménez, C.H., Eguía Salinas, I.: Demanda y oferta de educación superior: Integración total de la cadena de valor y las cadenas de suministro. Econ. y Adm. **2**(1) 21–50 (2017)
3. Sarrico, C.S., Rosa, M.J.: Supply chain quality management in education. Int. J. Qual. Reliab. Manag. **33**(4), 499–517 (2016)
4. Salazar, E., Capuz, S., De Reza, S., Padilla, J., Salinas, C.: Value stream mapping (VSM) for the process of professional formation. In: 17th International Congress Project Management Engineering, pp. 1387–1399, July 2013
5. Washington, A., Alfaro, D., Jonnathan, L., Rodríguez, S.U.: Tema: Aplicación De Lean VSM (Value Stream Mapping), UNIVERSIDAD ESTATAL DE MILAGRO (2018)
6. OCDE: Panorama de la educación 2019, Centro de México (2019). https://www.oecd.org/centrodemexico/estadisticas/. Accessed 21 Feb 2020
7. Trina Contreras, J.C.: Búsqueda de alternativas para la formación docente en la cuarta revolución industrial en el contexto universitario. Reforma Siglo XXI, vol. 100, pp. 46–49 (2019)
8. Habib, M.M., Hasan, I.: Supply chain management (SCM) - is it value addition towards academia? IOP Conf. Ser. Mater. Sci. Eng. **528**(1), 1–9 (2019)
9. Murali Krishna, M., Subbaiah, V.K.: Supply chain management: the educational organization perspective. ASIAN J. Manag. Res. **3**(1), 277–281 (2012)
10. Habib, M.: An integrated educational supply chain management (ITESCM). Ph.D. dissertation Graduate School of Information Technology, Assumption University of Thailand (2009)
11. Habib, M.: An empirical research of ITESCM (integrated tertiary educational supply chain management) model. In: Management and Services, October 2011
12. Briner, R.B., Denyer, D., Rousseau, D.M.: Evidence-based management: concept cleanup time? Academy of Management Perspective, p. 22, November 1996
13. Cigolini, R., Cozzi, M., Perona, M.: A new framework for supply chain management. Int. J. Oper. Prod. Manag. **24**(1), 7–41 (2004)
14. Owusu-Bio, M.K., Manso, J.F., Adiwokor, E.: Mapping the internal supply chain for educational institutions. A case study of Kwame Nkrumah University of Science and Technology. Eur. J. Bus. Manag. **7**(32), 32–42 (2015). http://www.iiste.org
15. Forero, D.E., Ramos, J.C.: La integración vertical en la cadena de abastecimiento de las instituciones de educación superior en Colombia, Criterio Libr. no. 22, p. 255 (2015)

16. Gopalakrishnan, G.: How to apply academic supply chain management: the case of an international university. Management **20**(1), 207–221 (2015)
17. Fajardo, S.A.D.: Rediseño de la Cadena de Suministro en función del tiempo de entrega, Universidad Autónoma de Nuevo León (2018)
18. Basu, G., Jeyasingam, J., Habib, M.M.: Education supply chain management model to achieve sustainability in private Universities in Malaysia: a review. Int. J. Supply Chain Manag. **5**(4), 24–37 (2017)
19. Melnyk, S.A., Narasimhan, R., DeCampos, H.A.: Supply chain design: issues, challenges, frameworks and solutions. Int. J. Prod. Res. **52**(7), 1887–1896 (2014)
20. Asmussen, J.N., Kristensen, J., Wæhrens, B.V.: Cost estimation accuracy in supply chain design: the role of decision-making complexity and management attention. Int. J. Phys. Distrib. Logist. Manag. **48**(10), 995–1019 (2018)
21. Rashid, S., Weston, R.: Design of an integrated methodology for analytical design of complex supply chains. Adv. Decis. Sci. **2012** (2012)
22. Báez Olvera, M.D.L.Á.: Apoyo a la decisión para el diseño y la planeación integrados de una cadena de suministro. Universidad Autónoma de Nuevo León (2015)
23. Rashid, S., Masood, T., Weston, R.H.: Unified modelling in support of organisation design and change. Proc. Inst. Mech. Eng. **223**, 055–1078 (2009)
24. Stewart, G.: Supply chain operations reference model, pp. 1–976 (2017)
25. Wang, W.Y.C., Chan, H.K., Pauleen, D.J.: Aligning business process reengineering in implementing global supply chain systems by the SCOR model. Int. J. Prod. Res. **48**(19), 5647–5669 (2010)
26. Prakash, S., Sandeep Gunjan, S., Rathore, A.: Supply chain operations reference (SCOR) model: an overview and a structured literature review of its application. In: International Conference on Smart Technologies for Mechanical Engineering, pp. 1–20, October 2013
27. Kersten, W., Saeed, M.A.: A SCOR based analysis of simulation in supply chain management. In: Proceedings - 28th European Conference on Modelling Simulation, ECMS 2014, pp. 461–469 (2014)
28. Bauer, D., Göbl, M.: Flexibility measurement issues in supply chain management. J. Appl. Leadersh. Manag. **5**, 1–14 (2017)
29. Gonzalez, V., Lozano, S.M.F., Sandoval, W.E.G., Villacreses, K.B., Vera, D.S.: Modelo del mapeo del flujo de valor - Value stream mapping (VSM) para la mejora de procesos de producción de empresa de Dulcería-café. In: Proceedings of LACCEI International Multi-conference on Engineering Educational Technology, vol. 2018-July, January 2018
30. Carrera, M.R., Sanchez, J.L.: ean Manufacturing La evidencia de una necesidad (2010)
31. Morlock, F., Meier, H.: Service value stream mapping in industrial product-service system performance management. Procedia CIRP **30**, 457–461 (2015)
32. Busse, C., Schleper, M.C., Weilenmann, J., Wagner, S.M.: Extending the supply chain visibility boundary: utilizing stake-holders for identifying supply chain sustainability risks. Int. J. Phys. Distrib. Logist. Manage. **47**(1), 18–40 (2017)
33. Carvalho, H., Barroso, A.P., MacHado, V.H., Azevedo, S., Cruz-Machado, V.: Supply chain redesign for resilience using simulation. Comput. Ind. Eng. **62**(1), 329–341 (2012)
34. Rivera, J.C.: El uso de la simulación para apoyar la toma de decisiones organizacionales. Rev. Estud. Adm. Empres. **9**(1), 70–84 (2016)
35. Brintrup, A., et al.: Supply chain data analytics for predicting supplier disruptions: a case study in complex asset manufacturing. Int. J. Prod. Res. **58**(11), 3330–3341 (2020)

36. Frantz, T.L., Carley, K.M., Wallace, W.A.: Computational organization theory. Encyclopedia of Operational Research Management Science, pp. 246–252 (2013)
37. Rodríguez-Fernández, Y., Abreu-Ledón, R., Franz, M.: Mapeo del Flujo de Valor para el análisis de sostenibilidad en cadenas de suministro agro-alimentarias. Ing. Ind. **40**(3), 316–328 (2019). [1]
38. Faulkner, W., Templeton, W., Gullett, D.: Visualizing sustainability performance of manufacturing systems using sustainable value stream mapping (SUS-VSM). In: International Conference on Industrial Engineering Operational Management, Istanbul, Turkey (2012)

Teaching of TCP Fundamental Operations Using a Digital Tool

Ilse Alicia López-Pedroza and Francisco de Asís López-Fuentes[✉]

Department of Information Technology, Universidad Autónoma Metropolitana - Cuajimalpa,
Av. Vasco de Quiroga 4871, Cuajimalpa, 05348 México City, Mexico
ilsepedrozaa1@gmail.com, flopez@cua.uam.mx

Abstract. Today, digital tools play an important role in education. These tools are a support to strengthen the knowledge of students while for teachers it can become part of their work material. Using digital didactic tools, the students can understand an algorithm with a certain degree of difficulty. We present in this paper a digital tool to support the teaching and learning of transmission control protocol (TCP) fundamental operations. Using interactive examples and animations, our didactic tool provides complementary information that help to understand the TCP basic concepts.

Keywords: Didactic software · Networking · TCP protocol · Simulation

1 Introduction

During the year 2020 the world has faced a pandemic that kept us in social confinement, this includes the fact that schools have been closed for a long period. However, in this situation, alternatives were sought that could help distance learning. The main resource used to meet these needs have been digital tools and video conferences. The importance of technologies in education has been reflected, even increasing their price at the market and worldwide level. A greater benefit could be seen in education, some teachers realized that these technological resources could be used in face-to-face classes or for homework. The importance of didactic tools in teaching is reflected worldwide, it has already been accepted as a complement to the information given by teachers or as the means of teaching where teachers take the resources as the main source for their classes. A teaching tool helps support inside or outside the classroom, as it is easy to access and intuitive. However, the main limitation faced the digital tools based on internet is access to the internet since several localities still do not have the necessary internet infrastructure.

Networking courses are an important core of different bachelor curriculum related to information technology and computer engineering. However, motivating students to learn topics related to networking such as internet protocols can be often difficult and boring mainly due because its theoretical subjects. In this work, we present a digital tool to support the teaching/learning process of the fundamental operations of the Transmission

J. A. Marmolejo-Saucedo et al. (Eds.): COMPSE 2020, LNICST 359, pp. 231–241, 2021.
https://doi.org/10.1007/978-3-030-69839-3_16

Control Protocol (TCP) [1]. Using this tool, we expect that students can acquire, reinforce, and exercise their knowledge about this important protocol. Interactive examples and animations are used to guide the user through this tool.

The rest of this work has the following organization. Section 2 presents information related to protocols and networking didactic tools. In Sect. 3 information about basic and fundamental aspects of TCP are described. In this section, we also explain the TCP basic operations to be implemented in our didactic tool. Section 4 presents the general design of our didactic tool, while its implementation is described in Sect. 5. Section 6 describes the tests and evaluations done to our tool. The article concludes in Sect. 7.

2 Related Work

Networking protocols are described in many textbooks [2–6], and its applications have been discussed extensively in the computer networking literature [7, 8]. In this section, we review some didactic tools related to our work presented in this paper. Authors in [9] present NEO as a web tool where communication protocols can be learned. This tool mainly shows detailed definitions about communication protocols. There are animation sections where are shown the characteristics and operations of each OSI/ISO and TCP layer reference models. Isiunne is proposed in [10] as a methodology for the development of teaching/learning tools using animations. This tool has simple animations, which are used to explain data communication concepts, the ISO/OSI reference model and data communication protocols. Its design has been planned for different user profiles as administrator, teacher, or student. Isiunne contains evaluations of the concepts shown, which are administered depending on the user profile with which it is entered. Kiva Network simulator (KivaNS) is proposed in [11] as a free and open source java-based application. KivaNS allows user to design data network schemes and to simulate the IP routing through these networks. Thus, we can find data network diagrams and packet routing simulations. KivaNS is mainly oriented to simulate the IP behavior, and emulates the basic operation of technologies in the link layer as Ethernet. The main objective of this tool is to help to design and understand the data networks operations, specifically the packets routing in the TCP/IP architecture, without needing a real infrastructure and traffic analysis tools. Other digital tools related to teaching of computer networks can be found in the literature, however most of these tools still have many characteristics to be covered and improved.

3 TCP Background

The Transport Control Protocol (TCP) is a protocol in the transport layer, and its main task is the reliable transportation of data through the network [2]. This protocol allows to exchange information between computers and application programs. TCP ensures that the transferred data arrive correctly, secure and in order. Main attributes of TCP are [2]:

- a fully duplex bidirectional virtual circuit.
- data is transmitted as a data stream.
- its reliable data transmission is based on:

- sequence numbers
- checksum
- acknowledgements
- retransmission when an acknowledgement is received timeout.
- greater efficiency based the sliding-window principle.
- urgent data and push function
- graceful connection shutdown
- transport-user addressing using port number.

The TCP protocol header has different fields with the following significance [2], [5]: *source and destination port number*, are fields of 16-bits and denote the initial and end points of a virtual circuit. The *sequence number* is a 32-bits word which refers to the send direction. The *acknowledge number* also is a 32-bits word and it applies to the number of bytes received by the other end [2]. The *data offset* contains the length of the TCP header. The *flags* are bits used to trigger actions in TCP. There are six flag bits in the TCP header, and one or more of them can be activated at the same time [2]:

1. URG - pointer in *Urgent* field is valid.
2. ACK - acknowledgment number is valid.
3. PSH - the receiver should pass this data to the application as soon as possible.
4. RST - resetting of the connection.
5. SYN - synchronize sequence numbers to initiate a connection.
6. FIN – the sender shutdowns the connection, and the data flow is finished.

The *window* contains the number of bytes that a receiver can accept in its data buffer for this connection. This field is used to control the data flow. The *checksum* includes a code which is used in the receiver to detect some error in transmission. The *urgent pointer* points to a data byte called urgent data which must be read immediately. The *options* field is used to add extra facilities not covered by the regular header.

The TCP protocol contains many functions which ensure that the data arrives correctly. For example, TCP establish a successful and secure connection to ensure that information is not lost. The main functions to be considered in our didactic tool are TCP connection establishment (normal case), retransmission and sliding window. In the following we give a briefly description of these functions.

3.1 TCP Connection Establishment

A TCP connection is established through an agreement of three. One side waits for a connection while the other side executes the connection. For this connection, protocol needs to specify the address, the port number, the TCP maximum segment size to be accepted, and optionally some user data. After this, transmitter waits for the response. The segment arrives at the receiver and it checks if there is any process in the list. Depending on what is on the list, the connection is rejected or accepted. If the connection is accepted, then a confirmation segment is returned, otherwise a reject response is sent to the transmitter. A SYN segment consumes 1 byte of sequence space [5]. Figure 1 shows how a TCP connection is established.

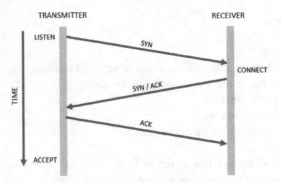

Fig. 1. Establishing a TCP connection.

3.2 Retransmission

During the information transmission may be loss of packets. Therefore, the retransmission is the way to ensure that the packets arrive correctly to its destination. TCP returns an ACK each time it receives data, on that path a timer is started. If the timer expires before the ACK arrives then the packet sending process is performed again. We can have n number of retransmissions, but all depends on the amount of lost packet that exist during the transmission. We can see this in Fig. 2.

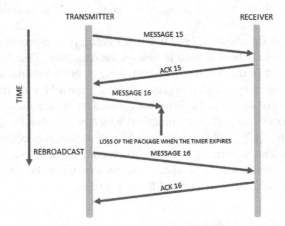

Fig. 2. An example of retransmission.

3.3 Sliding Window

TCP uses a sliding window scheme for data flow control in packet communications. Transmitter may send the number of bytes specified in the windows, without having to wait for an acknowledgement from the other part [2]. The sliding window can be enlarged or reduced depending on the needs. The aim is to carry the complete information from one side to the other. Figure 3 shows an example of how this function in the TCP protocol is done.

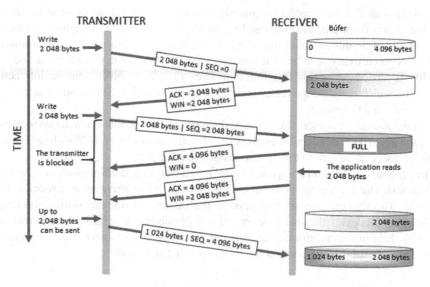

Fig. 3. An example of sliding window (adapted from [5]).

4   Analysis and Design

Designing an interface simple and easy-to-use both students and teachers is one of the objectives of this work. When a web page is created, we need to develop a system which should be easy to access and use by the main actors. In our case main actors are the students and teachers. This section describes the different design stages of our didactic tool.

4.1   System Structure

To develop our system, we have structured the TCP information into a main page, where each TCP function is represented. When the users enter the system, they can access all the information or only information that they could consider of interest. This is done through a main menu where the users can visualize this information.

4.2   Main Page

The main page shows the TCP definition and general information about this protocol. There is also a glossary with some technical terms that are used throughout the system. The main page of the system has a menu with three different options: TCP connection establishment, retransmission, and sliding window.

4.3 TCP Connection Establishment, Retransmission, and Sliding Window Sections

Any section in the main menu (connection establishment, retransmission or sliding window) has two options: definition and example. When the definition option is selected, we find a brief definition about the selected function and an animation. The animation shows a concrete example of how the function is performed between two devices and how the flow is carried out by this TCP function. The example option contains an interactive animation which represents a realistic case of how selected TCP function works (e.g.: connection establishment).

From these sections users can navigate through all the information in the system, they can learn about TCP connection establishment, retransmission or TCP sliding window. Even the users can return to the definitions or the examples.

In general, our design is proposed to use more images and animations avoiding use a lot of text. The animations invite to the user putting more attention in a specific TCP function. Thereby, our tool tries to capture the interest of students during the teaching/learning process. Likewise, teachers have a possibility to reinforce the knowledge given by them in the classroom. An approach based on animations can also be used to give repeated explanations about a topic or as a self-taught tool.

5   Implementation

Our didactic tool has been mainly developed using HTML and CSS language. Power Point and Scratch were used for the animations and examples. We use HTML to develop the system structure, the main menu was developed to display a submenu which shows the different options (definition and example) for each TCP function. We use CSS to define the colors and the fonts. Figure 4 shows the main page of the system where we can see at the top of menu the TCP functions (Our system has been written in Spanish).

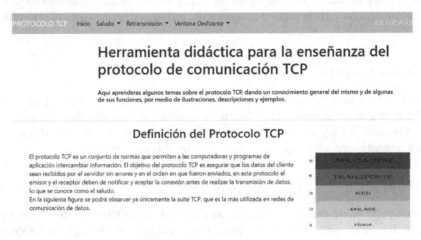

Fig. 4. System main page.

For a better understanding of the TCP, our system uses simple animations instead of images, since these animations explain step by step the processes of the TCP functions. First, the animations were made in Power Point, later they were integrated into the system using the iSpring tool. Using Power Point, we can draw the figures, add movements and more visual effects that help to understand the subject. We can obtain simple, understandable, and easy-to-use animations which can be viewed, stopped, restarted, or advanced. In this way, the user can see our tool as a more interactive method instead of an images-only collection. The Fig. 5 shows this animation development process and its final display in the system.

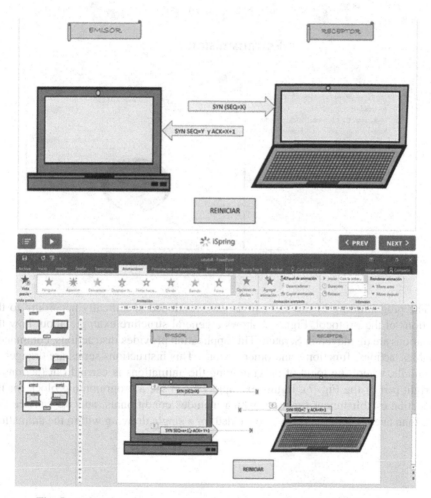

Fig. 5. Animation development for the connection establishment function.

The examples shown in the system are interactive, in the form of a game. So, the user can enter different data and simulate the moment when a failure in the function occurs or whether the function works correctly. Scratch [12] was used to develop the interactive examples. Scratch is a visual programming language, and it is an alternative to develop the examples in such a way that the general expectations of the system are met. The examples were programmed within the Scratch home page, so these examples can be accessed from this home page. Later the examples were added to the system. The examples can be reproduced as many times as the user wishes. Each time the user clicks on the green flag, the example will be started from the beginning, requesting the login data again. Figure 6 shows an example of how an interactive example for the retransmission function is displayed in the system.

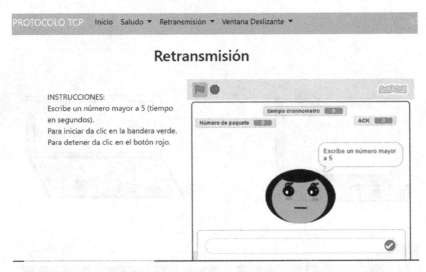

Fig. 6. Example of the retransmission function.

The programming of the animations was developed specifically according to the functions of the protocol. Figure 7 shows a general structure example about how the animations are displayed in Scratch. This application provides instructions, commands, variables, actions, functions, and other options. This instructions series are dragged to the middle, where the logic of programming the animations is carried out (actions in the right part of the Fig. 7). In this example we can see a programming block for the connection establishment function, which includes conditionals, and we can see that more than one block has already been added for a single drawing within the animation.

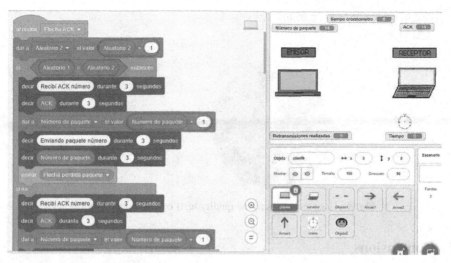

Fig. 7. Scratch development for the retransmission function.

6 Evaluation

Our didactic tool was tested with some users to evaluate its performance. The users have previous knowledge of TCP, some them are students and other graduates. Therefore, not all have recent knowledge over this protocol.

Users had access to the system, later they were given to fill out a form where the main questions were to highlight the design of the system and how this information was useful to them. The responses were very homogeneous since most of them had the same observations and likes for the system. The profile of the users who were tested was users with previous knowledge of TCP. The tests applied to users yielded results that helped to assess the quality of the system as well as see the advantages and improvements that can be made to it in the future work.

In general, the system was liked by the users. However, the design part received the most observations. The users made several observations related to the design and placing a greater emphasis on font size and system colors. Regarding the evaluation of the system, we observe that users showed a greater acceptance for the animations and interactive examples than the text. Some users did not use the text, because they were guided by the examples and animations. In fact, some users did not use the text, because they were guided by the examples and animations. Some results of our evaluation are shown in the Fig. 8.

¿Qué información te fue más útil?

8 respuestas

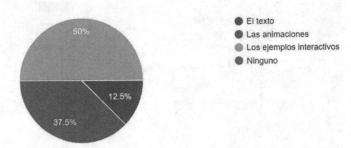

El texto
Las animaciones
Los ejemplos interactivos
Ninguno

Fig. 8. User responses to the quality tests of our didactic tool.

7 Conclusions

The current world situation has shown us the importance of information technology, especially in education. In this paper, we present a didactic tool for teaching TCP protocol, which shows how information technology can play an important role in the teaching and learning process. The TCP protocol, like other subjects, can be taught through computational means such as cellular phones or electronic tablet. In our proposed didactic tool, we have learned that visual aspects are very important. The inclusion of little texts helps the users to have more taste and ease for learning of a subject. Our tool does not try to substitute to the teacher, but it tries to complement the information about TCP. Likewise, our tool could help to the students to clarify doubts related to TCP. Our didactic tool is easily accessible, it can be consulted within classrooms, at home or anywhere with internet access. A limitation of our tool is its dependence of internet because it cannot be used in location where the internet access is not available.

As future work, our didactic tool can be extended in different aspects. For example, we can add more animations, more extensive examples, new evaluation questionnaires, or aspect related to usability can be considered. Also, an open access version for teachers or students could improve this tool with feedback or collaboration. Finally, others TCP functions can be added such as round-trip time during the retransmission or a comparison with UDP communication protocol.

References

1. Postel, J.: Transmission Control Protocol. RFC 793 (1981)
2. Santifaller, M.: TCP/IP and NFS Internetworking in UNIX environment, Addison-Wesley (1981)
3. Peterson, L.L., Davie, B.S.: Computer Networks: A Systems Approach. 5th edition, Morgan Kaufmann (2011)
4. Kurose, J., Ross, K.: Computer Networking: A Top-Down Approach. 7th edition, Pearson (2016)
5. Tanenbaum, A., Wetherall, D.J.: Computer Networks. 5th edition, Pearson (2011)
6. Comer, D.E.: Computer Networks and Internet. 1st edition, Prentice-Hall (1997)

7. Stalling, W.: Data and computer communications. 8th edition, Pearson Prentice Hall (2007)
8. Comer, D.E., Stevens D.L.: Internetworking TCP/IP Vol. 2, 3th edition, Prentice-Hall (1995)
9. NEO: http://neo.lcc.uma.es/evirtual/cdd/tutorial/Indice.html. Accessed 08 Dec 2019
10. Isiunne: http://www.lsiunne.com.ar/_. Accessed 10 Dec 2019
11. KivaNS: http://www.disclab.ua.es/kiva/. Accessed 10 Dec 2019
12. Scratch: https://scratch.mit.edu/. Accessed 22 Jul 2020

Author Index

Printed in the United States
By Bookmasters